Ultimate 2021
FLORIDA & FEDERAL MPJE REVIEW

MASTERING THE MPJE COMPETENCIES

GARY CACCIATORE, Pharm.D., J.D.

Published by Dr. C's Review Guides
www.mpjereviews.com
info@mpjereviews.com

January 2021

© 2021 Gary Cacciatore. All rights reserved. No part of this publication may be reproduced, stored in a database or retrieval system, or transmitted in any form or by any means electronic, mechanical, photocopying, recording, or otherwise without written permission of the publisher.

VIOLATION OF COPYRIGHT WILL RESULT IN LEGAL ACTION, INCLUDING CIVIL AND CRIMINAL PENALTIES.
The consent of the publisher does not extend to copying for general distribution, for promoting, for creating new works, or for resale. Specific permission must be obtained in writing from Dr. C's Review Guides.

Trademark Notice: Product or corporate names may be trademarks or registered trademarks and are used only for identification and explanation, without intent to infringe.

ISBN 978-0-578-79449-5

CONTENTS

1	Introduction
3	About the Author
5	Acronyms
7	Information on the Multistate Pharmacy Jurisprudence Exam (MPJE®)
11	MPJE® Competency Statements from the NAPLEX®/MPJE® Candidate Registration Bulletin

19	**CHAPTER ONE**	Federal Food, Drug, and Cosmetic Act (FDCA), Poison Prevention Packaging Act (PPPA), and Other Miscellaneous Federal Laws
21	Federal Food, Drug, and Cosmetic Act (FDCA) and Major Amendments
28	Prohibited Acts Under the FDCA
31	Other Provisions of the FDCA and Federal Regulations
42	Poison Prevention Packaging Act of 1970 (PPPA)
45	Other Federal Laws and Regulations
48	Privacy—HIPAA and HITECH

53	**CHAPTER TWO**	Federal Controlled Substances Act (FCSA) and Florida Controlled Substances Act (FLCSA) and Applicable Rules
55	Drug Classification
58	Scheduling of Compounded Controlled Substances
59	Registration
63	Ordering and Transferring Controlled Substances
69	Additional Requirements for Controlled Substances
79	Dispensing Controlled Substance Prescriptions
89	Schedule II Prescriptions
97	Schedule III–V Prescriptions
99	Methadone, Opiate Dependence, Naloxone, and Methamphetamine Controls
104	E-FORCSE™: The Florida Prescription Drug Monitoring Program (PDMP)

109	**CHAPTER THREE** | Florida Laws—Part 1 Overview, Prescriptive Authority, Board of Pharmacy, Definitions, and Licensure
111	Florida Laws Impacting Pharmacy Practice
112	Prescriptive Authority and Scope of Practice
121	Florida Board of Pharmacy (§ 465.004)
123	Definitions
127	Licensure of Individuals
138	Pharmacy Permits
146	Florida Food Drug and Cosmetic Act—Chapter 499
153	**CHAPTER FOUR** | Florida Pharmacy Law—Part 2 Pharmacy Personnel and Pharmacy Practice
155	Laws and Rules Applicable to Individuals
160	Laws and Rules for All Pharmacy Permits or Applicable to Pharmacists in Any Location
173	Pharmacists Order For Medicinal Drugs, Drug Therapy Management, Collaborative Practice, & Test and Treat
184	Community Pharmacies
200	Institutional Pharmacies
210	Nuclear Pharmacies and Nuclear Pharmacists
213	**CHAPTER FIVE** | USP Chapters and Compounding Laws and Rules
215	Introduction to USP Chapters
217	USP 797 Pharmaceutical Compounding—Sterile Preparations
227	USP 800 Hazardous Drugs—Compounding in Healthcare Settings
237	Florida Rules on Compounding
247	**CHAPTER SIX** | Disciplinary Actions and Procedures, and Miscellaneous Laws and Rules
249	Disciplinary Actions and Procedures
261	Miscellaneous Laws and Rules

265	**CHAPTER SEVEN** | Summary Charts and Self-Assessment Questions	
267	Summary Chart of Days' Supply Limitations	
268	Summary Chart of Notification, Reporting, and Other Time-Limited Requirements	
270	Self-Assessment Questions	
285	Explanatory Answers	

INTRODUCTION

Dr. C's Ultimate Florida and Federal MPJE® Review 2021 provides an overview of state and federal law impacting the practice of pharmacy in Florida. Although primarily intended to serve as a study guide for the Florida Multistate Pharmacy Jurisprudence Exam (MPJE®), the book also serves as an excellent reference book on Florida pharmacy law by reorganizing and summarizing the statutes and rules in a more comprehensible manner.

The book includes explanatory notes to help the reader make sense of often confusing or ambiguous statutory and rule language, and groups different rules and statutes together based on subject matter to better facilitate learning. **Study Tips** are provided throughout the book to note important material and help clarify information that is often misunderstood or causes confusion.

As you experienced when you were a pharmacy student, recent graduate, or a seasoned pharmacist who last sat for an exam more than a few years ago, your study plan and preparation are critical to your success. The Florida MPJE requires you to fully comprehend state and federal laws, regulations, and a pharmacist's responsibilities.

Dr. C's Ultimate Florida and Federal MPJE® Review has been developed by a pharmacy regulatory expert with education and experience in both law and pharmacy. The book is designed to assist you in focusing on the elements of the exam that may appear on the Florida MPJE, although the author has no specific knowledge of questions that are on the exam. All references to sections of statute refer to the Florida Pharmacy Act (FPA) unless otherwise specified.

The key to success is to allow adequate time in your study plan to review parts of the law that are least familiar to you. We believe this book will help in the process and support your successful exam completion.

*MPJE is a registered trademark of the National Association of Boards of Pharmacy

ABOUT THE AUTHOR

Gary Cacciatore, Pharm.D., J.D.

Gary Cacciatore lives in Houston, Texas, and currently serves as Associate Regulatory Counsel and Vice President of Regulatory Affairs for Cardinal Health, Inc., a global, integrated healthcare services and products company, providing customized solutions for hospitals, health systems, pharmacies, ambulatory surgery centers, clinical laboratories, and physician offices worldwide.

Prior to joining Cardinal Health, Dr. Cacciatore was an Assistant Professor at the University of Houston College of Pharmacy and the University of Houston Law Center, where he taught courses in pharmacy law and ethics, drug information, and food and drug law. He currently serves as an Adjunct Associate Professor at the University of Houston College of Pharmacy, teaching the pharmacy law course, and as an Adjunct Associate Professor at the University of Florida College of Pharmacy.

Dr. Cacciatore is the coauthor of *Texas and Federal Pharmacy and Drug Law*, a comprehensive textbook used by nearly all of the pharmacy schools in Texas, and *The Ultimate Texas MPJE Review Guide*, the leading Texas MPJE review book, which has been utilized by pharmacists and students from all 50 states and 10 foreign countries. He is also the author of *Dr. C's Ultimate Federal Pharmacy Law Review*.

Dr. Cacciatore received his Doctor of Pharmacy degree with high honors from the University of Florida College of Pharmacy. He earned his Doctor of Jurisprudence degree with honors from the University of Houston Law Center. He is a past President of the American Society for Pharmacy Law (ASPL), and in 2015, he received the Joseph L. Fink III Founders Award from ASPL for outstanding and sustained contributions to the professions of pharmacy and law. Dr. Cacciatore was named the Outstanding Alumnus by the University of Florida College of Pharmacy for 2021.

Dr. Cacciatore is admitted to the bar in Texas and is a registered pharmacist in Texas and Florida.

ACRONYMS

Most acronyms are defined the first time they are used in this book (and often several times), but here is a list of some of the major acronyms used:

ACPE	Accreditation Council for Pharmacy Education
APRN	Advanced Practice Registered Nurse
ASC	Ambulatory Surgical Center
CE	Continuing Education
CEU	Continuing Education Unit
CFR	Code of Federal Regulations
cGMP	current Good Manufacturing Practices
DBPR	Department of Business and Professional Regulation (Florida)
DDDC	Division of Drugs, Devices and Cosmetics (Florida)
DEA	Drug Enforcement Administration
FAC	Florida Administrative Code (Rules)
FBOP	Florida Board of Pharmacy
FCSA	Federal Controlled Substances Act
FDA	Food and Drug Administration
FDCA	Food, Drug, and Cosmetic Act (Federal)
FDLE	Florida Department of Law Enforcement
FFDCA	Florida Food, Drug, and Cosmetic Act
FLCSA	Florida Controlled Substances Act
FPA	Florida Pharmacy Act
GMP	Good Manufacturing Practices
HIPAA	Health Insurance Portability and Accountability Act
LTCF	Long Term Care Facility
MPJE	Multistate Pharmacy Jurisprudence Exam
NABP	National Association of Boards of Pharmacy
NAPLEX	North American Pharmacist Licensure Exam
NDC	National Drug Code
OTC	Over-the-counter
PA	Physician Assistant
PDM	Prescription Department Manager
PDMP	Prescription Drug Monitoring Program
PIC	Pharmacist-in-charge
PPI	Patient Package Insert
PPPA	Poison Prevention Packaging Act
PRN	Professional Recovery Network
REMS	Risk Evaluation and Mitigation Strategies
USP	United States Pharmacopeia

Information on the Multistate Pharmacy Jurisprudence Exam (MPJE®)

General Information

Registration Bulletin

Detailed information on the MPJE is available from the National Association of Boards of Pharmacy (NABP) NAPLEX/MPJE Registration bulletin, which is available for download at NABP's website. The bulletin contains detailed information on registering for the exam, scheduling testing appointments, fees, identification requirements, security, question types, score results, and most importantly the competency statements (see below). Candidates should download and read the registration bulletin carefully.

Exam Content and Structure

The MPJE is a 120-item computer-based examination that uses adaptive technology. This means the computer adapts the questions you receive based on your previous responses. You are allowed 2 and 1/2 hours to complete the exam. You must complete 107 questions for your exam to be scored. Of the 120 items on the exam, 100 count toward your score. The questions not counting toward your score are being pretested; however, you will not know which questions count toward your score and which questions are being pretested. Because it is a computer-based examination, you cannot go back and review a question or change an answer once you have confirmed it and moved to the next question. You also cannot skip a question. Since there is a penalty for unanswered questions, you should answer all the questions.

The exam content and questions are developed by Board of Pharmacy representatives, practitioners, and educators from around the country who serve as item writers. Each state Board of Pharmacy approves the questions that are used for its particular state.

You must achieve a score of 75 to pass the exam. This is not 75%, but a scaled score whereby your performance is measured against predetermined minimum abilities. The maximum score is 100.

While you must have a good base knowledge of the laws and rules governing the practice of pharmacy in your state, simply memorizing the laws will not suffice. The exam is not simply questions that ask you to identify or repeat the law. There are many situational questions that will require you to apply the law to the facts provided. These types of questions are not as easy. When approaching these types of questions, it is helpful to remember that the goal of the Board of Pharmacy is to protect the public health. Answers that address that goal are most likely to be correct. At the same time, the Board of Pharmacy must also enforce the laws, so many of the laws and rules are intended to assist the Board with that function. Rules related to recordkeeping and documentation are especially important to boards of pharmacy to help them identify who or what caused an error in a pharmacy that may cause patient harm. Keeping these functions of the boards of pharmacy in mind may help you when trying to choose between answers on the exam. The MPJE consists of several types of questions, including multiple choice, multiple response (i.e., select all that apply), and ordered response. When the MPJE began using multiple response questions, they no longer needed to write multiple choice questions that were K-type questions. K-type questions are multiple choice questions where the answer choices consist of different combinations of the available choices. For example, choice A is I only, choice B is I and III, choice C is II and IV, and choice D is I, II, and III. Although new questions on the MPJE are not K-type questions, there are likely still many older questions that are K-type questions, so you should not be surprised to see these types of questions. Examples of each question type are provided below:

Multiple Choice Sample Question

A Florida pharmacist must obtain how many continuing education (CE) hours to renew his or her license in each renewal period?

a. 15 hours
b. 20 hours
c. 30 hours
d. 40 hours

Multiple Response Sample Question

Which are permissible ways for a pharmacist to obtain continuing education? Select all that apply.

____ Completing an ACPE accredited continuing education course
____ Attending a Board of Pharmacy meeting at which disciplinary hearings are conducted
____ Auditing a course at a College of Pharmacy
____ Performing volunteer services to the indigent within the state

STUDY TIP: When answering multiple response questions, it is recommended that you choose more than one answer. If only one answer is correct, it is more likely to be a multiple choice question.

Ordered Response Sample Question

Place the following products in order from the least abuse potential to the greatest abuse potential. (All options must be used.) Left-click the mouse to highlight, drag, and order the answer options.

Unordered Options	Ordered Response
Tylenol with Codeine	_____
Sudafed	_____
Valium	_____
Vicodin	_____

STUDY TIP: Make sure you read the ordered response question carefully and put the items in the correct order, not the reverse order. Double-check the order before hitting the Submit button.

Federal Versus State Law

When comparing federal law versus state law, the general rule is you always follow the stricter law. In the rare instance where state and federal law directly conflict so that you cannot follow one without violating the other, the federal law would prevail. It is important to understand that **no distinction is made on the MPJE exam between federal and state law questions**. You should answer each question in terms of the prevailing laws of the state in which you are seeking licensure, which for purposes of this book is Florida.

This means that you should not see a question on the exam that starts out with the words "According to the Federal Controlled Substances Act . . ." Such a question would not be valid because it is asking you to answer the question based on federal law only. If Florida has a law that is different and stricter than the federal law, that is the law that must be followed and would be the correct answer.

Pre-MPJE

NABP offers a Pre-MPJE exam that candidates can register to take online at NABP's website. This is the only practice exam that features valid questions from previous versions of the MPJE. The exam consists of 40 questions, and 50 minutes are allotted to complete the exam. The Pre-MPJE can be taken only one time for each jurisdiction a person is seeking licensure in. The official NABP Pre-MPJE exam can only be taken on the NABP's website. There are other websites using the term "Pre-MPJE" that are not affiliated with NABP.

MPJE Competency Statements

Each question on the MPJE is tied to a specific competency statement. You must master a certain number of competencies to pass the exam. It is possible that you will have to answer more than one question correctly in order to pass a particular competency, depending on the difficulty of the questions. So you may see more than one question on a single topic. In addition, you may get a similar question or questions from the same competency because one or more of those questions are being pretested and do not count toward your score. It is imperative that you read through the competency statements in the registration bulletin, although not every competency statement is covered under Florida law. The MPJE® Competency Statements have been reprinted on the following pages.

MPJE®
Competency Statements
from the
NAPLEX®/MPJE® Candidate Registration Bulletin

Area 1 | Pharmacy Practice (83%)

1.1 **Legal responsibilities of the pharmacist and other pharmacy personnel**

1.1.1 Unique legal responsibilities of the pharmacist-in-charge (or equivalent), pharmacists, interns, and pharmacy owners

Responsibilities for inventory, loss and/or theft of prescription drugs, the destruction/disposal of prescription drugs, and the precedence of Local, State, or Federal requirements

1.1.2 Qualifications, scope of duties, and conditions for practice relating to pharmacy technicians and all other non-pharmacist personnel

Personnel ratios, duties, tasks, roles, and functions of non-pharmacist personnel

1.2 **Requirements for the acquisition and distribution of pharmaceutical products, including samples**

1.2.1 Requirements and record keeping in relation to the ordering, acquiring, and maintenance of all pharmaceutical products and bulk drug substances/excipients

Legitimate suppliers, pedigrees, and the maintenance of acquisition records

1.2.2 Requirements for distributing pharmaceutical products and preparations, including the content and maintenance of distribution records

Legal possession of pharmaceutical products (including drug samples), labeling, packaging, repackaging, compounding, and sales to practitioners

1.3 **Legal requirements that must be observed in the issuance of a prescription/drug order**

1.3.1 Prescription/order requirements for pharmaceutical products and the limitations on their respective therapeutic uses

Products, preparations, their uses, and limitations applicable to all prescribed orders for both human and veterinary uses

1.3.2 Scope of authority, scope of practice, and valid registration of all practitioners who are authorized under law to prescribe, dispense, or administer pharmaceutical products, including controlled substances

Federal and State registrations, methadone programs, office-based opioid treatment programs, regulations related to retired or deceased prescribers, internet prescribing, and limits on jurisdictional prescribing

1.3.3 Conditions under which the pharmacist participates in the administration of pharmaceutical products or in the management of patients' drug therapy

Prescriptive authority, collaborative practice, consulting, counseling, medication administration (including immunizations and vaccines), ordering labs, medication therapy management, and disease state management

1.3.4 Requirements for issuing a prescription/order

Content and format for written, telephonic voice transmission, electronic facsimile, computer and internet, during emergency conditions, and tamper-resistant prescription forms

1.3.5 Requirements for the issuance of controlled substance prescriptions/orders

Content and format for written, telephonic voice transmission, electronic facsimile, computerized and internet, during emergency conditions, conditions for changing a prescription, time limits for dispensing initial prescriptions/drug orders, and requirements for multiple Schedule II orders

1.3.6 Limits of a practitioner's authority to authorize refills of a pharmaceutical product, including controlled substances

1.4 **Procedures necessary to properly dispense a pharmaceutical product, including controlled substances, pursuant to a prescription/drug order**

1.4.1 Responsibilities for determining whether prescriptions/orders were issued for a legitimate medical purpose and within all applicable legal restrictions

Corresponding responsibility, maximum quantities, restricted distribution systems, red flags/automated alerts, controlled substances, valid patient/prescriber relationship, and due diligence to ensure validity of the order

1.4.2 Requirements for the transfer of existing prescription/order information from one pharmacist to another

1.4.3 Conditions under which a prescription/order may be filled or refilled

Emergency fills or refills, partial dispensing of a controlled substance, disaster or emergency protocol, patient identification, requirement for death with dignity, medical marijuana, and conscience/moral circumstances

1.4.4 Conditions under which prospective drug use review is conducted prior to dispensing

Patient-specific therapy and requirements for patient-specific documentation

1.4.5 Conditions under which product selection is permitted or mandated

Consent of the patient and/or prescriber, passing-on of cost savings, and appropriate documentation

1.4.6 Requirements for the labeling of pharmaceutical products and preparations dispensed pursuant to a prescription/order

Generic and therapeutic equivalency, formulary use, auxiliary labels, patient package inserts, FDA medication guides, and written drug information

1.4.7 Packaging requirements of pharmaceutical products, preparations, and devices to be dispensed pursuant to a prescription/order

Child-resistant and customized patient medication packaging

1.4.8 Conditions under which a pharmaceutical product, preparation, or device may not be dispensed

Adulteration, misbranding, and dating

1.4.9 Requirements for compounding pharmaceutical products

Environmental controls, release checks and testing, beyond use date (BUD), and initial and ongoing training

1.4.10 Requirements for emergency kits

Supplying, maintenance, access, security, and inventory

1.4.11 Conditions regarding the return and/or reuse of pharmaceutical products, preparations, bulk drug substances/excipients, and devices

Charitable programs, cancer or other repository programs, previously dispensed, and from "will call" areas of pharmacies

1.4.12 Procedures and requirements for systems or processes whereby a non-pharmacist may obtain pharmaceutical products, preparations, bulk drug substances/excipients, and devices

Pyxis (vending), after-hour's access, telepharmacies, and secure automated patient drug retrieval centers

1.4.13 Procedures and requirements for establishing and operating central processing and central fill pharmacies

Remote order verification

1.4.14 Requirements for reporting to PMP, accessing information in a PMP, and the maintenance of security and confidentiality of information accessed in PMPs

1.4.15 Requirements when informed consent must be obtained from the patient and/or a duty to warn must be executed

Collaborative practice and investigational drug therapy

1.5 **Conditions for making an offer to counsel or counseling appropriate patients, including the requirements for documentation**

1.5.1 Requirements to counsel or to make an offer to counsel

1.5.2 Required documentation necessary for counseling

1.6 **Requirements for the distribution and/or dispensing of nonprescription pharmaceutical products, including controlled substances**

1.6.1 Requirements for the labeling of nonprescription pharmaceutical products and devices

1.6.2 Requirements for the packaging and repackaging of nonprescription pharmaceutical products and devices

1.6.3 Requirements for the distribution and/or dispensing of poisons, restricted, nonprescription pharmaceutical products, and other restricted materials or devices

Pseudoephedrine, dextromethorphan, emergency contraception, and behind-the-counter products, as appropriate

1.7 **Procedures for keeping records of information related to pharmacy practice, pharmaceutical products, and patients, including requirements for protecting patient confidentiality**

1.7.1 Requirements pertaining to controlled substance inventories

1.7.2 Content, maintenance, storage, and reporting requirements for records required in the operation of a pharmacy

Prescription filing systems, computer systems and backups, and prescription monitoring programs

1.7.3 Requirements for protecting patient confidentiality and confidential health records

HIPAA requirements and conditions for access and use of information

1.8 **Requirements for handling hazardous materials such as described in USP 800**

1.8.1 Requirements for appropriate disposal of hazardous materials

1.8.2 Requirements for training regarding hazardous materials

Reverse distributors, quarantine procedures, comprehensive safety programs, and Material Safety Data Sheets

1.8.3 Environmental controls addressing the proper storage, handling, and disposal of hazardous materials

Ventilation controls, personal protective equipment, work practices, and reporting

1.8.4 Methods for the compounding, dispensing, and administration of hazardous materials

All hazardous materials including sterile and non-sterile compounding

Area 2 | Licensure, Registration, Certification, and Operational Requirements (15%)

2.1 **Qualifications, application procedure, necessary examinations, and internship for licensure, registration, or certification of individuals engaged in the storage, distribution, and/or dispensing of pharmaceutical products (prescription and nonprescription)**

2.1.1 Requirements for special or restricted licenses, registration, authorization, or certificates

Pharmacists, pharmacist preceptors, pharmacy interns, pharmacy technicians, controlled substance registrants, and under specialty pharmacist licenses (Nuclear, Consultant, etc.)

2.1.2 Standards of practice related to the practice of pharmacy

Quality assurance programs (including peer review), changing dosage forms, therapeutic substitution, error reporting, public health reporting requirements (such as notification of potential terrorist event, physical abuse, and treatment for tuberculosis), and issues of conscience and maintaining competency

2.1.3 Requirements for classifications and processes of disciplinary actions that may be taken against a registered, licensed, certified, or permitted individual

2.1.4 Requirements for reporting to and participating in programs addressing the inability of an individual licensed, registered, or certified by the Board to engage in the practice of pharmacy with reasonable skill and safety

Impairment caused by the use of alcohol, drugs, chemicals, or other materials, or mental, physical, or psychological conditions

2.2 **Requirements and application procedure for the registration, licensure, certification, or permitting of a practice setting or business entity**

2.2.1 Requirements for registration, license, certification, or permitting of a practice setting

In-state pharmacies, out-of-state pharmacies, specialty pharmacies, controlled substance registrants, wholesalers, distributors, manufacturers/repackagers, computer services providers, and internet pharmacies

2.2.2 Requirements for an inspection of a licensed, registered, certified, or permitted practice setting

2.2.3 Requirements for the renewal or reinstatement of a license, registration, certificate, or permit of a practice setting

2.2.4 Classifications and processes of disciplinary actions that may be taken against a registered, licensed, certified, or permitted practice setting

2.3 Operational requirements for a registered, licensed, certified, or permitted practice setting

2.3.1 Requirements for the operation of a pharmacy or practice setting that is not directly related to the dispensing of pharmaceutical products

Issues related to space, equipment, advertising and signage, security (including temporary absences of the pharmacist), policies and procedures, libraries, and references (including veterinary), and the display of licenses

2.3.2 Requirements for the possession, storage, and handling of pharmaceutical products, preparations, bulk drug substances/excipients, and devices, including controlled substances

Investigational new drugs, repackaged or resold drugs, sample pharmaceuticals, recalls, and outdated pharmaceutical products

2.3.3 Requirements for delivery of pharmaceutical products, preparations, bulk drug substances/excipients, and devices, including controlled substances

Issues related to identification of the person accepting delivery of a drug, use of the mail, contract delivery, use of couriers, use of pharmacy employees, use of kiosks, secure mailboxes, and script centers, use of vacuum tubes, and use of drive-up windows

Area 3 | General Regulatory Processes (2%)

3.1 Application of regulations

3.1.1 Laws and rules that regulate or affect the manufacture, storage, distribution, and dispensing of pharmaceutical products, preparations, bulk drug substances/excipients, and devices (prescription and nonprescription), including controlled substances

Food, Drug, and Cosmetic Act(s) and Regulations, the Controlled Substances Act(s) and Regulations, OBRA 90's Title IV Requirements, Practice Acts and Rules, other statutes and regulations, including, but not limited to, dispensing of methadone, child-resistant packaging, tamper-resistant packaging, drug paraphernalia, drug samples, pharmacist responsibilities in Medicare-certified skilled-nursing facilities, NDC numbers, and schedules of controlled substances

CHAPTER ONE

Federal Food, Drug, and Cosmetic Act (FDCA), Poison Prevention Packaging Act (PPPA), and Other Miscellaneous Federal Laws

CHAPTER ONE
Federal Food, Drug, and Cosmetic Act (FDCA), Poison Prevention Packaging Act (PPPA), and Other Miscellaneous Federal Laws

I. **Federal Food, Drug, and Cosmetic Act (FDCA) and Major Amendments**
   A. Food, Drug, and Cosmetic Act of 1938
      1. Following deaths caused by sulfanilamide elixir in 1937, Congress passed the first legislation that required new drugs to be proven safe prior to marketing.
      2. Established the FDA and is the primary federal law dealing with food, drug, cosmetic, and medical device safety today (with many amendments).
   B. Durham-Humphrey Amendment of 1951
      1. Established two classes of drugs: prescription and over-the-counter (OTC).

STUDY TIP: You are expected to know those pharmaceutical products that require a prescription. It is particularly important to know that certain products in the same drug class may be either prescription or nonprescription depending on the product or the strength. For example, some insulin products are non-prescription; however, certain other insulin products such as Lantus® and Humalog® are prescription-only products. Another example is that ibuprofen 400 mg, 600 mg, and 800 mg products require a prescription while ibuprofen 200 mg products do not.

BONUS STUDY TIP: Medical oxygen is also a prescription drug; however, under Florida law it may be supplied to a patient by a medical oxygen retail establishment licensed by the Florida Department of Business and Professional Regulation (DBPR) pursuant to a valid prescription. It is one of the few drugs in Florida that can be dispensed by a business that does not have a pharmacy permit.

      2. Authorized verbal prescriptions and prescription refills.
   C. Kefauver-Harris Amendments of 1962
      1. Required new drugs be proven safe and effective for their claimed use. Prior to this amendment, new drugs only had

to be safe. This amendment required new drugs to also be effective for their stated use.
2. Increased safety requirements for drugs and established Good Manufacturing Practices (GMPs) for manufacturing of drugs.
3. Gave FDA jurisdiction over prescription drug advertising.

D. Prescription Drug Marketing Act of 1987 (PDMA)
1. Bans the re-importation of prescription drugs and insulin products produced in the United States (except by the manufacturer).

Note: This prohibition is on the re-importation of drugs produced in the United States and then exported. This is different than the importation of drugs manufactured in another country. Importation of drugs is generally prohibited; however, the Medicine Equity and Drug Safety (MEDS) Act of 2000 and the Medicare Prescription Drug Improvement and Modernization Act of 2003 both have provisions that allow importation of drugs under specific conditions. One of those conditions is that the Secretary of Health and Human Services (HHS) must certify to Congress that such imports do not threaten the health and safety of the American public and provide cost savings. FDA finalized new rules on importation on September 24, 2020, which permit states to serve as sponsors to import drugs from Canada under certain conditions. A few states (including Florida) have passed laws to allow drug importation from Canada, but as of the date of publication of this book, no state plan has been approved by HHS. See also Florida International Pharmacy Permit in Chapter 3, Section VI. E.5.

2. Bans the sale, trade, or purchase of prescription drug samples.

STUDY TIP: The Florida Food, Drug and Cosmetic Act (§ 499.028) and rules on samples are consistent with federal law, but make a distinction between drug samples and "starter packs." Starter packs or "initial dose packs" or "stock samples" are human prescription drugs that are generally distributed without charge by manufacturers or distributors to pharmacies to be placed in stock and sold at retail. Although starter packs are generally given without charge to the pharmacy, they are not intended to be a free sample to the consumer, nor are they labeled as such. Starter packs are subject to regulation as prescription drugs in the same manner as stock shipments of prescription drugs. Starter packs are not drug samples.

3. Mandates the storage, handling, and recordkeeping requirements for prescription drug samples.
    a. These include obtaining written requests for samples from practitioners and requiring signatures of practitioners upon receipt.
    b. Samples may only be provided to practitioners or, upon request of a licensed practitioner, to an institutional pharmacy or to pharmacies of other healthcare facilities.
    c. Community pharmacies should not possess prescription drug samples, except for prescription drugs that may be ordered by a pharmacist. The only exception to this would be a community pharmacy that is part of a healthcare entity such as a community pharmacy owned by a hospital.
    d. In Florida, a Complimentary Drug Distributor Permit from the Division of Drugs, Devices and Cosmetics (DDDC) of the Department of Business and Professional Regulation (DBPR) is required to hold, distribute, and dispose of prescription drug samples.

STUDY TIP: Samples are mentioned four times in the MPJE Competency Statements. The primary thing to remember is that a community pharmacy that is not affiliated with a healthcare entity may not be in possession of prescription drug samples.

4. Prohibits, with certain exceptions, the resale of prescription drugs purchased by hospitals or healthcare facilities.
   Note: This is intended to prevent diversion of drugs due to price diversion because hospitals generally receive lower prices for drugs than community pharmacies.
E. The Drug Quality and Security Act (DQSA) of 2013—These amendments to the FDCA addressed two primary topics: large-scale compounding by pharmacies and establishment of a framework for a uniform track-and-trace system for prescription drugs throughout the supply chain to prevent counterfeit drugs.
    1. Drug Compounding Quality Act (DCQA).
        a. Passed in response to an outbreak of fungal meningitis in over 20 states in the fall of 2012, which was traced to a contaminated injectable steroid produced by the New England Compounding Center. This outbreak resulted

in the death of over 60 patients and over 750 cases of infection.
   b. Outsourcing facilities, often referred to as 503B facilities, are permitted to compound sterile products without receiving patient-specific prescriptions or medication orders. They are primarily regulated by FDA and are subject to FDA's current Good Manufacturing Practices (cGMPs).
   Note: Despite this law being passed in 2013, there are currently only approximately 70 registered outsourcing facilities in the entire country.

STUDY TIP: Florida requires in-state outsourcing facilities to obtain a Special Sterile Compounding Permit and out-of-state outsourcing facilities to obtain a Nonresident Sterile Compounding Outsourcing Facility Permit. *See Chapter 2*

   c. Compounding pharmacies that are not registered with FDA as an "outsourcing facility" are often referred to as 503A facilities or 503A pharmacies and may only compound products pursuant to an individual prescription or medication order. They are permitted to do limited anticipatory compounding, are primarily regulated by the states, and are subject to USP Chapter 797 quality standards for sterile compounding.
   d. Outsourcing facilities that meet the Act's requirements are exempt from the premarket approval requirements for new drugs (FDCA Section 505), adequate directions for use requirements (FDCA Section 502(f)(1)), and drug track-and-trace provisions (FDCA Section 582).
   Note: Outsourcing facilities are not exempt from good manufacturing practices.
   e. Outsourcing facilities must:
      (1) Have a licensed pharmacist who provides direct oversight over the drugs compounded;
      (2) Register as an outsourcing facility. The FDA website provides a list of the names of each outsourcing facility, along with the state where the facility is located, whether the facility compounds from bulk drug substances, and whether drugs compounded from bulk are sterile or nonsterile;

- (3) Report to the Secretary of HHS upon registering, and every six months thereafter, the drugs sold in the previous six months;
- (4) Be inspected by FDA according to a risk-based inspection schedule and pay annual fees to support it;
- (5) Report serious adverse event experiences within 15 days and conduct a follow-up investigation and reporting similar to current drug manufacturers; and
- (6) Label products with a statement identifying them as a compounded drug and other specified information about the drug.

f. Outsourcing facilities may not compound a drug product that includes a bulk drug substance unless:
- (1) The bulk drug substance appears on a list identifying bulk drug substances for which there is a clinical need (the 503B bulks list); or
- (2) The drug product compounded from such bulk drug substance appears on FDA's drug shortage list at the time of compounding, distribution, and dispensing.

Note: FDA issued an Interim Policy on Compounding Using Bulk Drug Substances under Section 503B of the FDCA. See the compounding section of FDA's website for more information.

STUDY TIP: FDA has issued several additional guidance documents to implement the Compounding Quality Act that are beyond the scope of this book. Detailed information may be found at FDA's website.

2. Drug Supply Chain Security Act (DSCSA) (Track and Trace).
   a. Provides for a uniform national framework for an electronic track-and-trace system for prescription drugs as they move through the supply chain, and sets national standards for states to license drug wholesaler distributors.
   b. Applies to prescription drugs for human use in finished dosage form, but certain products are exempted, including blood and blood components, radioactive drugs, imaging drugs, certain intravenous products for fluid replacement, dialysis solutions, medical gases,

compounded drugs, medical convenience kits containing drugs, certain combination products, sterile water, and products for irrigation.
  c. Manufacturers are required to provide "Transaction Data" for each product sold, and pharmacies are required to receive transaction data and pass this information along if they further distribute the product.
  d. "Transaction Data" includes Transaction Information, Transaction History, and a Transaction Statement.
     (1) Transaction Information includes the product's name, strength, and dosage form; NDC number; container size and number of containers; date of transaction; and name and address of the person from whom ownership is being transferred and to whom ownership is being transferred. A unique product identifier or serialized numerical identifier (SNI) will also be required that identifies an individual bottle or unit of sale.
     (2) Transaction History is a paper or electronic statement that includes prior transaction information for each prior transaction back to the manufacturer.
     (3) Transaction Statement is a paper or electronic statement by the seller that the seller is authorized (licensed), received the product from an authorized (licensed) person, received the transaction information and transaction history from the prior owner if required, did not knowingly ship a suspect or illegitimate product, has systems and processes to comply with verification requirements, and did not knowingly provide false transaction information.
  e. Pharmacies must investigate and properly handle suspect and illegitimate products.
     (1) Suspect products are products that one has reason to believe are potentially counterfeit, diverted, stolen, subject to a fraudulent transaction, intentionally adulterated, or appear otherwise unfit for distribution such that they would result in serious adverse health consequences or death to humans.
     (2) Illegitimate products are products for which credible evidence shows that the products are counterfeit, diverted, stolen, subject of a fraudulent transaction,

intentionally adulterated, or appear otherwise unfit for distribution such that they would result in serious adverse health consequences or death to humans.
- (3) Pharmacies must investigate any suspect or illegitimate product. As part of the investigation, a pharmacy must verify the product identifier of at least 3 products or 10% of the suspect product, whichever is greater, or all of the packages if there are fewer than 3. Pharmacies must also verify any illegitimate product in response to a notification of illegitimate product from FDA or a trading partner.
Note: This requirement was scheduled to go into effect on November 23, 2020, but FDA has delayed enforcement until November 23, 2023.
- (4) If a product is illegitimate, pharmacies must notify FDA using Form FDA 3911 and notify trading partners within 24 hours. Pharmacies should also work with the manufacturer to prevent an illegitimate product from reaching patients.

f. Pharmacies that are "distributing" (distributing is defined as providing a drug to anyone other than the consumer/patient, as compared to dispensing, which is providing a drug to the patient/consumer) must have a wholesale distribution license and must pass DSCSA transaction data with that distribution. The only exceptions to having a distribution license and passing transaction data are as follows:
- (1) When the distribution is between two entities that are affiliated or under common ownership;
- (2) When a dispenser is providing product to another dispenser on a patient-specific basis;
- (3) When a dispenser is distributing under emergency medical reasons; or
- (4) When a dispenser is distributing "minimal quantities" to a licensed practitioner for office use.

g. Other provisions of the DSCSA will be implemented gradually, eventually requiring electronic tracking and tracing of product at the individual package level using a unique product identifier on each package, by 2023.

II. Prohibited Acts Under the FDCA

Nearly all violations of the FDCA cause the products to be adulterated and/or misbranded. It is important to understand the difference between these two concepts. Although drug manufacturers are more likely to violate the FDCA, actions taken by pharmacists (e.g., a dispensing error) could also cause a product to be adulterated or misbranded. It is likely these are the types of situations that may be covered on the MPJE.

A. Adulteration—A drug is adulterated if:
1. It contains any filthy, putrid, or decomposed substance.
2. It has been prepared or held under insanitary conditions where it may have been contaminated.
3. The methods of manufacture do not conform to current good manufacturing practices (cGMPs).
4. It has been manufactured, processed, packed, or held in any factory, warehouse, or establishment and the owner, operator, or agent of such factory, warehouse, or establishment delays, denies, or limits an inspection, or refuses to permit entry or inspection.
5. The container is composed of any poisonous or deleterious substance which may contaminate the drug.
6. It contains an unsafe color additive.
7. It purports to be a drug in an official compendium and its strength differs from or its quality or purity falls below the compendium standard, unless the difference is clearly stated on the label.
    Note: This means that if the product claims to meet USP standards and its strength or quality does not meet those standards, it is adulterated.
8. It is not in a compendium, and its strength differs from or its quality falls below what it represents.
    Note: This means that even if the product does not claim to meet USP standards, if the strength or quality differs or falls below what is stated on its label or labeling, it is adulterated.
9. It is mixed or packed with any substance that reduces its strength or quality, or the drug has been substituted in whole or in part.

STUDY TIP: If a product's strength is less than what is represented on its label, it could be both misbranded and adulterated. See C. below.

B. Misbranding—A drug is misbranded if:
1. The labeling is false or misleading in any particular way.
2. It is a prescription drug and the manufacturer's labeling fails to contain the following information:
   a. The name and address of the manufacturer, packer, or distributor.
   b. Brand and/or generic name of the drug or drug product.
   c. The net quantity (weight, quantity, or dosage units).
   d. The weight of active ingredient per dosage unit.
   e. The federal legend, "Rx only."
   f. If not taken orally, the specific routes of administration (e.g., for IM injection).
   g. Special storage instructions, if appropriate.
   h. Manufacturer's control number (lot number).
   i. Expiration date.
   j. Adequate information for use. For prescription drugs, this is the package insert and medication guide or patient package insert if required. This also includes other information required (e.g., certain products, including opioids and benzodiazepines, require "black box warnings" to alert healthcare professionals about essential information regarding the product).

STUDY TIP: These labeling requirements are for the manufacturer's container. When a pharmacist dispenses a drug to a patient pursuant to a valid prescription, the label does not have to contain all of these elements. State prescription labeling requirements would dictate what is required on the label.

3. It is an OTC drug and fails to contain the following:
   a. A principal display panel, including a statement of identity of the product.
   b. The name and address of the manufacturer, packer, or distributor.
   c. Net quantity of contents.
   d. Cautions and warnings needed to protect user.
   e. Adequate directions for safe and effective use (for layperson).
   f. Content and format of OTC product labeling in "Drug Facts" panel format, including:
      (1) Active Ingredients.
      (2) Purpose.

(3) Use(s)—indications.
(4) Warnings.
(5) Directions.
(6) Other Information.
(7) Inactive Ingredients (in alphabetical order).
(8) Questions? (optional) followed by telephone number.
4. It is a drug liable to deterioration unless it is packaged or labeled accordingly.
5. The container is made, formed, or filled as to be misleading.
6. The drug is an exact imitation of another drug or offered for sale under the name of another drug.
7. It is dangerous to health when used in the dosage or manner suggested in the labeling.
8. It is packaged or labeled in violation of the Poison Prevention Packaging Act.

STUDY TIP: Pharmacists do not usually concern themselves with these labeling requirements as it is expected that manufacturers will label their products appropriately, but you should know the labeling requirements for OTC drugs.

C. Adulteration and Misbranding as Applied to Pharmacies
1. Dispensing a prescription without authorization causes the drug to be misbranded even if it is labeled correctly by the pharmacist. This is because a prescription drug product is only exempt from the manufacturer's labeling requirements in B. 2. above when it is dispensed pursuant to a valid prescription.
2. Misfilling a prescription with the wrong drug, strength, or directions for use will always cause the drug to be misbranded.
3. If a misfilled prescription involves the wrong strength of the drug prescribed, it would also be adulterated. This is because the definition of adulteration includes when the strength differs from or quality falls below that which it represents.
4. If a drug is subject to a Risk Evaluation and Mitigation Strategy (REMS) and it is prescribed or dispensed without meeting the requirements of the REMS, it is misbranded because the REMS program is part of the official labeling of the drug.
5. The advertising or promotion of a compounded drug that is false or misleading would be misbranding.

6. An expired drug product in a manufacturer's bottle is adulterated because after the expiration date, the strength cannot be assured. If a prescription is filled using an expired product, it may also be misbranded if the pharmacist placed a beyond-use date that is after the expiration date of the drug.

STUDY TIP: You are more likely to encounter questions related to adulteration and misbranding based on scenarios in a pharmacy.

III. **Other Provisions of the FDCA and Federal Regulations**
   A. Special Warning Requirements for OTC Products in the FDCA

STUDY TIP: These are special labeling requirements under federal regulations for products containing these ingredients. Normally the manufacturer's label would include these warnings, but you should be familiar with these requirements.

1. FD&C Yellow No. 5 (tartrazine) and No. 6 (21 CFR 201.20)—Must disclose presence and provide warning in "precautions" section of label that may cause allergic reaction in certain susceptible persons.
2. Aspartame (21 CFR 201.21)—Must contain warning in "precautions" section of labeling to the following effect: Phenylketonurics: Contains phenylalanine __ mg per (dosage unit).
3. Sulfites (21 CFR 201.22)—Prescription drugs containing sulfites (often used as a preservative) must contain an allergy warning in the "warnings" section of the labeling.
4. Mineral Oil (21 CFR 201.302)—Requires warning to only be taken at bedtime and not be used in infants unless under advice of a physician. Label also cannot encourage use during pregnancy.
5. Wintergreen Oil (methyl salicylate) (21 CFR 201.303 and 201.314(g)(1))—Any drug containing more than 5% methyl salicylate (often used as flavoring agent) must include warning that any use other than directed may be dangerous and that the article should be kept out of reach of children.
6. Sodium Phosphates (21 CFR 201.307)—Limits the amount of sodium phosphates oral solution to not more than 90 ml per OTC container. Also requires specific warnings.

7. Isoproterenol inhalation preparations (21 CFR 201.305)—Requires warning not to exceed dose prescribed and to contact physician if difficulty in breathing persists.
8. Potassium Salt Preparations for Oral Ingestions (21 CFR 201.306)—Requires warning regarding nonspecific small-bowel lesions consisting of stenosis, with or without ulceration, associated with the administration of enteric-coated thiazides with potassium salts.
9. Ipecac Syrup (21 CFR 201.308)
    a. The following statement (boxed and in red letters) must appear: "For emergency use to cause vomiting in poisoning. Before using, call physician, the poison prevention center, or hospital emergency room immediately for advice."
    b. The following warning must appear: "Warning: Keep out of reach of children. Do not use in unconscious persons."
    c. The dosage of the medication must appear. The usual dosage is 1 tablespoon (15 ml) in individuals over 1 year of age.
    d. May only be sold in 1 oz. (30 ml) containers.
10. Phenacetin (acetophenetidin) (21 CFR 201.309)—Must contain warning about possible kidney damage when taken in large amounts or for a long period of time.
11. Salicylates (21 CFR 201.314)—Aspirin and other salicylate drugs must have special warnings for use in children, including warning regarding Reye's syndrome. Retail containers of 1 1/4 grain (pediatric) aspirin cannot be sold in containers holding more than 36 tablets.
12. OTC Drugs for Minor Sore Throats (21 CFR 201.315)—Any OTC product label that states "For the temporary relief of minor sore throats" must include this warning: "Warning—Severe or persistent sore throat or sore throat accompanied by high fever, headache, nausea, and vomiting may be serious. Consult physician promptly. Do not use more than 2 days or administer to children under 3 years of age unless directed by physician."
13. Alcohol Warning (21 CFR 201.322)—Internal analgesics and antipyretics, including acetaminophen, aspirin, ibuprofen, naproxen, ketoprofen, etc., are required to have a warning for persons consuming 3 or more alcoholic beverages per day and to consult with a doctor before taking.

14. Over-the-counter drugs for vaginal contraceptive and spermicide use containing nonoxynol 9 as the active ingredient (21 CFR 201.325)—Are subject to several warning requirements, including "Sexually transmitted diseases (STDs) alert: This product does not protect against HIV/AIDS or other STDs and may increase the risk of getting HIV from an infected partner."
15. OTC Pain Relievers (21 CFR 201.326)
   a. Acetaminophen.
      (1) Must have "acetaminophen" prominently displayed.
      (2) Must warn about liver toxicity.
      (3) Must warn not to use with other products containing acetaminophen and to talk to a doctor or pharmacist before taking with warfarin.
   b. Nonsteroidal Anti-inflammatory Drugs (NSAIDs).
      (1) Must include term "NSAID" prominently on label.
      (2) Must contain "stomach bleeding" warning.
16. OTC Products Containing Iron in Solid Oral Dosage Form (21 CFR 310.518(a))
   a. Must provide the following warning: "Accidental overdose of iron-containing products is a leading cause of fatal poisoning in children under 6. Keep this product out of reach of children. In case of accidental overdose, call a doctor or poison control center immediately."
   b. This warning requirement also applies to dietary supplements containing iron through 21 CFR 101.17(e).
   c. FDA previously had a rule that required unit-dose packaging for iron-containing dietary supplements and drug products that contain 30 milligrams (mg) or more of iron per dosage unit, but that rule was eliminated based on a court case in 2003 that concluded FDA did not have the authority to pass such a rule.

B. Additional OTC Requirements
1. Tamper-Evident Packaging—Manufacturers and packagers of OTC drugs (except dermatological, dentifrice, insulin, or lozenge products) for sale at retail must package products in a tamper-evident package.
2. Repackaging of OTC Products—A pharmacist that repackages OTC products would be subject to cGMP requirements and would have to meet all additional requirements, including tamper-evident packaging, if offered for sale to the public.

STUDY TIP: If a patient wishes to purchase an OTC drug in a smaller package size than what is commercially available, a pharmacist cannot break open a commercial OTC product and sell the lesser quantity by placing it in a vial and labeling it. The only way this can be done is if the patient has a prescription for the smaller quantity, and the OTC drug is filled as a prescription as discussed below.

    3. When an OTC product is prescribed and filled as a prescription, the OTC labeling requirements do not have to be followed. The prescription drug labeling requirements would apply and would include the prescriber's directions for use. If an OTC drug is filled as a prescription, any instructions for refills would apply as would beyond use dates (valid for one year).
- C. FDA Drug and Device Recall Classifications
  1. Class I—Reasonable probability product will cause either serious adverse effects on health or death.
  2. Class II—May cause temporary or medically reversible adverse effects on health or where probability of serious adverse effects is remote.
  3. Class III—Not likely to cause adverse health consequences.
- D. Advertising and Promotion of Prescription Drugs
  1. Prescription drug advertising is regulated by FDA.
  2. Over-the-counter (OTC) drug advertising is regulated by the Federal Trade Commission (FTC).
  3. Advertising of Prescription Drug Prices (including by pharmacists)—The advertising of prescription drug prices is considered reminder advertising under FDA regulations (21 CFR 200.200). However, such advertising is exempt from FDA advertising regulations provided that the following conditions are met:
     a. The only purpose of the advertising is to provide information on price, not information on the drug's safety, efficacy, or indications for use.
     b. The advertising contains the proprietary name of the drug (if any), the generic name of the drug, the drug's strength, the dosage form, and the price charged for a specific quantity of the drug.
     c. The advertising may include other information, such as the availability of professional or other types of services, as long as it is not misleading.

        d. The price stated in the advertising shall include all charges to the consumer; mailing and delivery fees, if any, may be stated separately.
Note: Florida law also prohibits pharmacies from advertising or promoting the sale of controlled substances. See Chapter 4. Section II. I.3.
   4. A pharmacy that compounds products may advertise that they provide compounding services, including that they compound specific products. However, if a pharmacy makes any therapeutic claims regarding those products, they would be subject to FDA's rules on advertising, which are complex and beyond the scope of this book.
E. Patient Package Inserts (PPIs)
   1. Supplied by the manufacturer and written for a layperson.
   2. Required to be given to patients when prescriptions for certain products are dispensed.
   3. Currently required for:
        a. Oral contraceptives (21 CFR 310.501).
        b. Estrogen-containing products (21 CFR 310.515).
   4. Hospitalized or institutionalized patients—A PPI must be provided to a patient prior to the first administration of the drug and every 30 days thereafter.

STUDY TIP: This probably does not happen in practice, but you need to know that it is technically required.

   5. Failure to provide a PPI for these drugs would cause them to be misbranded.
F. Medication Guides (MedGuides)
   1. Similar to PPI program but without requirements for institutionalized patients.
   2. FDA requires Medication Guides for drugs when:
        a. Patient labeling could prevent serious adverse effects.
        b. Product has serious risks relative to benefits.
        c. Patient adherence to directions is crucial.
   3. Medication Guides must be written in a standard format and in language suitable for patients.
   4. Manufacturers must obtain FDA approval before distributing Medication Guides and are responsible for ensuring that a sufficient number of Medication Guides are provided to pharmacies. Many manufacturers include the Medication

Guide at the bottom of the package insert, but most pharmacy computer systems also print Medication Guides for the products that need them at the time of dispensing.
  5. FDA maintains a searchable Medication Guide database on its website, and there are over 1,000 products that now require a Medication Guide. Some of the drugs, drug classes, and biologicals requiring Medication Guides include:
     a. Accutane® (isotretinoin)
     b. Antidepressants in children and teenagers
     c. Coumadin® (warfarin sodium)
     d. Epogen® (epoetin alfa)
     e. Forteo® (teriparatide, rDNA origin)
     f. Lindane® shampoo and lotion
     g. Lotronex® (alosetron hydrochloride)
     h. Nolvadex® (tamoxifen)
     i. Non-Steroidal Anti-Inflammatory Drugs (NSAIDs)
     j. Remicade® (infliximab)
     k. Trizivar® (abacavir sulfate, lamivudine, and zidovudine)
     l. Opioid analgesics and cough products
     m. Benzodiazepines
  6. Failure to provide a Medication Guide when dispensing a drug that requires one would cause the drug to be misbranded.
G. Risk Evaluation and Mitigation Strategies (REMS)
  1. REMS are strategies to manage a known or potential serious risk associated with a drug, drug class, or biological product. FDA requires a REMS if FDA finds that it is necessary to ensure that the benefits of the drug, drug class, or biological product outweigh the risks of the product. A REMS can include a Medication Guide, a Patient Package Insert, a communication plan, elements to assure safe use, and an implementation system. It must also include a timetable for assessment of the REMS.
  2. Elements to assure safe use may include:
     a. Special training, experience, or certification of healthcare practitioners prescribing the drugs;
     b. Special certification for pharmacies, practitioners, or healthcare settings that dispense the drug;
     c. Dispensing drugs to patients only in certain healthcare settings such as hospitals;

d. Dispensing drugs to patients with evidence or other documentation of safe use conditions, such as laboratory test results;
   e. Monitoring patients using the drug; or
   f. Enrolling each patient using the drug in a registry.
3. A complete list of products with approved REMS can be found on FDA's website and may include an entire drug class, such as the Opioid Analgesic REMS. I have included summaries of two of the most extensive REMS below, but you should be familiar with the most common REMS and which products are subject to a REMS.

STUDY TIP: Some REMS place requirements only on prescribers. You are more likely to be asked questions about REMS programs that place requirements on pharmacists.

4. Example REMS—Isotretinoin (Accutane) iPLEDGE Program
   a. Only doctors registered in iPLEDGE can prescribe isotretinoin. Doctors registered with iPLEDGE must agree to assume the responsibility for pregnancy counseling of female patients of childbearing potential. Prescribers must obtain and enter into the iPLEDGE system negative test results for those female patients of childbearing potential prior to prescribing isotretinoin.
   b. Only patients registered in iPLEDGE can be prescribed isotretinoin. In addition to registering with iPLEDGE, patients must comply with a number of key requirements that include completing an informed consent form, obtaining counseling about the risks and requirements for safe use of the drug, and, for women of childbearing potential, complying with required pregnancy testing and use of contraception.
   c. Only pharmacies registered in iPLEDGE can dispense isotretinoin. To register in iPLEDGE, a pharmacy must select a Responsible Site Pharmacist who must obtain iPLEDGE program information and registration materials via the internet (*www.ipledgeprogram.com*) or telephone (1-866-495-0654) and sign and return the completed registration form. To activate registration, the

Responsible Site Pharmacist must access the iPLEDGE program via the internet (*www.ipledgeprogram.com*) or telephone (1-866-495-0654) and attest to the following points:
- **(1)** I know the risk and severity of fetal injury/birth defects from isotretinoin.
- **(2)** I will train all pharmacists on the iPLEDGE program requirements.
- **(3)** I will comply and seek to ensure that all pharmacists comply with the iPLEDGE program requirements.
- **(4)** I will obtain isotretinoin from iPLEDGE-registered wholesalers.
- **(5)** I will return to the manufacturer (or delegate) any unused product.
- **(6)** I will not fill isotretinoin for any party other than a qualified patient.

d. To dispense isotretinoin, pharmacists must obtain authorization from iPLEDGE via the internet (*www.ipledgeprogram.com*) or telephone (1-866-495-0654) signifying the patient is registered, has received counseling and education, and is not pregnant.

e. Females of reproductive potential have a 7-day prescription window to get an isotretinoin prescription filled. This 7-day window starts with the pregnancy test specimen collection date, not the date of the result of the test.

f. Product is dispensed in blister packages that cannot be broken, and a 30-day supply is the maximum quantity that can be dispensed.

g. No refills are allowed.

5. Example REMS—Thalomid (thalidomide) REMS
   a. Prescriber Requirements
      - **(1)** The prescriber enrolls and becomes certified with Celgene for the Thalomid REMS program.
      - **(2)** The prescriber counsels patient on benefits and risks of Thalomid.
      - **(3)** The prescriber provides contraception and emergency contraception counseling.
      - **(4)** The prescriber verifies negative pregnancy test for all female patients of reproductive potential.

(5) The prescriber completes a Thalomid Patient-Physician Agreement Form with each patient and sends to Celgene.
   (6) The prescriber/patient completes applicable mandatory confidential survey.
   (7) The prescriber obtains an authorization number from Celgene and writes it on every prescription along with patient risk category.
   (8) The prescriber writes no more than a 4-week (28-day) supply, with no automatic refills or telephone prescriptions.
   (9) The prescriber sends Thalomid prescription to a certified pharmacy.
 b. Pharmacy Requirements
   (1) Pharmacy must be certified in the Thalomid REMs program with Celgene.
   (2) Prescriptions can only be accepted with an authorization number and patient risk category.
   (3) Authorization numbers are valid for 7 days from the date of the last pregnancy test for female of reproductive potential and 30 days from the date issued for other patients.
   (4) Pharmacy must obtain a confirmation number prior to dispensing via toll-free number or online. The confirmation number is valid for 24 hours and must be entered on the prescription. This means the prescription must be dispensed within 24 hours of obtaining the confirmation number.
   (5) No automatic refills or telephone prescriptions are permitted.
   (6) Prescription must be written for 4-week (28-day) supply or less.
   (7) No refills are allowed and subsequent prescriptions may be dispensed only if there are 7 days or less remaining on the existing prescription.
   (8) A certified Thalomid REMS counselor must counsel the patient, and counseling must be documented.
   (9) Prescription must be dispensed with a medication guide.
   (10) Prescriptions cannot be transferred to another pharmacy without prior authorization from Celgene.

H. National Drug Code (NDC) Number
  1. A unique 10-character number that identifies a particular drug by manufacturer or packager (labeler), product, and package size.
     a. First 4 to 5 digits = labeler code.
     b. Next 3 to 4 digits = specific drug, strength, dosage form.
     c. Last 1 to 2 digits = package size.
  2. NDC numbers are required for a drug manufacturer to list their product with FDA, and FDA suggests they be included on the drug's label, although it is not technically required. All drug manufacturers include an NDC number because they facilitate automated processing of drug data by government agencies, third-party payers, wholesalers, and manufacturers.

STUDY TIP: NDC numbers should not appear on non-drug products. If a dietary supplement or medical device has an NDC number on its label, it would be misbranded. Medical devices have unique device identifiers (UDIs) instead of NDC numbers. Any product that implies it is an FDA-approved drug when it is not would also be misbranded.

---

  3. While nearly all drug products have an NDC number, an NDC code does not indicate a drug is approved by FDA. There are some unapproved drugs that have NDC numbers.
  4. FDA has proposed to standardize the NDC format and move to an 11-digit code, but that proposed change has not yet been adopted.

I. FDA Orange Book
  1. Official name is *Approved Drug Products with Therapeutic Equivalence Evaluations*.
  2. Available at *http://www.fda.gov/cder/ob/*.
  3. The primary source for determining generic equivalency of drugs. To be considered generically equivalent, a drug must be both pharmaceutically equivalent and therapeutically equivalent to the reference drug product (normally the brand-name drug).
  4. Definitions
     a. Pharmaceutical equivalents are drug products in identical dosage forms and route(s) of administration that contain identical amounts of the identical active drug ingredient.

    b. Therapeutic equivalents are approved drug products that are pharmaceutical equivalents for which bioequivalence has been demonstrated, and they can be expected to have the same clinical effect and safety profile when administered to patients under the conditions specified in the labeling. *Note: This means the drug is bioequivalent to the reference drug product.*
5. Uses 2-letter coding system to indicate equivalency with first letter being the key:
   a. A = Drug products that the FDA considers to be pharmaceutically equivalent and therapeutically equivalent.
   b. B = Drug products that the FDA considers NOT to be pharmaceutically equivalent and therapeutically equivalent.

STUDY TIP: The first letter of the 2-letter code tells you if the product is considered equivalent. It is recommended that the reader look up an Orange Book listing in the FDA Orange Book database online and be familiar with its format.

6. Products with no known or suspected bioequivalence issues:
   a. AA—conventional dosage forms.
   b. AN—solutions and powders for aerosolization.
   c. AO—injectable oil solutions.
   d. AP—injectable aqueous solutions.
   e. AT—topical products.
7. Products with actual or potential bioequivalence problems, but for which adequate scientific evidence has established bioequivalence for those products, are given a rating of AB.

J. FDA Purple Book
1. Official name is *Lists of Licensed Biological Products with Reference Product Exclusivity and Biosimilarity or Interchangeability Evaluations.*
2. Lists biological products that are considered biosimilars and provides interchangeability evaluations for these products.
3. "Biosimilar" or "biosimilarity" means that the biological product is highly similar to the reference product, notwithstanding minor differences in clinically inactive components, and there are no clinically meaningful differences between the biological product and the reference product in terms of the safety, purity, and potency of the product.

4. An interchangeable product is a product that has been shown to be biosimilar to the reference product and can be expected to produce the same clinical result as the reference product in any given patient.
5. Only biological products that have been designated "interchangeable" may be substituted for the original reference product by a pharmacist.
Note: While there are several biosimilar products on the market (such as adalimumab, bevacizumab, and epoetin alfa), as of the date of publication of this book, FDA has not designated any of them as interchangeable.

IV. Poison Prevention Packaging Act of 1970 (PPPA)
A. Administered by Consumer Product Safety Commission.
B. Requires child-resistant containers for all prescription drugs and for the following nonprescription drugs, drug classes, preparations, or dietary supplements:
  1. Aspirin—Any aspirin-containing preparation for human use in dosage form intended for oral administration.
  2. Methyl salicylate (oil of wintergreen)—Liquid preparations containing more than 5% by weight of methyl salicylate unless packaged in pressurized spray containers.
  3. Controlled drugs—Any preparation for human use in a dosage form intended for oral administration that consists in whole or in part of any substance subject to control under the Federal Controlled Substances Act.
  Note: There are some Schedule V controlled substances available without a prescription under federal law. See Chapter 3
  4. Methyl alcohol (methanol)—Household substances in liquid form containing 4% or more by weight of methyl alcohol unless packaged in a pressurized spray container.
  5. Iron-containing drugs—With the exception of animal feeds used as vehicles for the administration of drugs, noninjectable animal and human drugs providing iron for therapeutic or prophylactic purposes, which contain a total amount of elemental iron equivalent to 250 mg.
  6. Dietary supplements containing iron—With the exception of those preparations in which iron is present solely as a colorant, dietary supplements that contain an equivalent of 250 mg or more of elemental iron in a single package.

7. Acetaminophen—Preparations for human use in a dosage form intended for oral administration and containing more than 1 g of acetaminophen in a single package.
   Exemptions:
   a. Acetaminophen-containing effervescent tablets or granules containing less than 10% acetaminophen with a median lethal dose greater than 5 g/kg of body weight and that release at least 85 ml of carbon dioxide per grain of acetaminophen when placed in water.
   b. Unflavored acetaminophen-containing preparations in powder form, other than those intended for pediatric use, that are packaged in unit doses with no more than 13 grains of acetaminophen per unit dose and that contain no other substance subject to the special packaging requirements.
8. Diphenhydramine HCl—Preparations for human use in oral dosage forms containing more than the equivalent of 66 mg of diphenhydramine base in a single package.
9. Ibuprofen—Preparations for human use in oral dosage forms containing 1 gram or more of ibuprofen in a single package.
10. Loperamide—Preparations for human use in oral dosage forms containing more than 0.045 mg of loperamide in a single package.
11. Lidocaine—Products containing more than 5 mg of lidocaine in a single package (includes all dosage forms, including creams, sprays, and transdermal patches).
12. Dibucaine—Products containing more than 0.5 mg of dibucaine in a single package (includes all dosage forms, including creams, sprays, and transdermal patches).
13. Naproxen—Preparations for human use in oral dosage forms containing 250 mg or more of naproxen in a single package.
14. Ketoprofen—Preparations for human use in oral dosage forms containing more than 50 mg of ketoprofen in a single package.
15. Fluoride—Products containing more than 50 mg of elemental fluoride and more than 0.5% fluoride in a single package.
16. Minoxidil—Preparations for human use containing more than 14 mg of minoxidil in a single package (includes topical products that must continue to meet requirements once applicator is installed by consumer).

17. Imidazolines—Products containing 0.08 mg or more in a single package. Imidazolines are a drug class that includes tetrahydrozoline, naphazoline, oxymetazoline, and xylometazoline often found in ophthalmic and nasal products.
18. Any drug switched from Rx to OTC status.

C. Exemptions:
1. Request of patient or physician.

STUDY TIP: Only the patient can provide a blanket request for all future prescriptions. The prescriber can only request a non-child-resistant container on an individual prescription. The request is not legally required to be in writing, although it is good practice to have it in writing.

---

2. Bulk containers not intended for household use.
3. Drugs distributed to institutionalized patients.
4. One package size of OTC drugs designed for the elderly.
5. Specific prescription and nonprescription drug exemptions include:
   a. Oral contraceptives, conjugated estrogens, and norethindrone acetate in manufacturer's dispenser package.
   b. Medroxyprogesterone acetate tablets.
   c. Sublingual nitroglycerin and sublingual and chewable isosorbide dinitrate of 10 mg or less.
   d. Aspirin and acetaminophen in effervescent tablets or granules.
   e. Potassium supplements in unit-dose packaging.
   f. Sodium fluoride containing not more than 264 mg of sodium fluoride per package.
   g. Anhydrous cholestyramine and colestipol packets.
   h. Erythromycin ethylsuccinate granules for oral suspension and oral suspensions in packages containing not more than 8 g of erythromycin.
   i. Erythromycin ethylsuccinate tablets in packages containing no more than 16 g of erythromycin.
   j. Prednisone tablets containing no more than 105 mg per package.
   k. Methylprednisolone tablets containing no more than 84 mg per package.
   l. Mebendazole tablets containing no more than 600 mg per package.

    m. Betamethasone tablets containing no more than 12.6 mg per package.
    n. Preparations in aerosol containers intended for inhalation.
    o. Pancrelipase preparations.
    p. Sucrose preparations in a solution of glycerol and water.
    q. Hormone replacement therapy products that rely solely upon the activity of one or more progestogen or estrogen substances.

STUDY TIP: It is important to know all of the products that are exempt from the Poison Prevention Packaging Act, including details as to strengths and dosage forms.

V. Other Federal Laws and Regulations
  A. Federal Hazardous Substances Act of 1966
    1. The Consumer Product Safety Commission administers and enforces this Act, which is intended to protect consumers from hazardous and toxic substances.
    2. Requires the label on the immediate package of a hazardous product and any outer wrapping or container that might cover up the label on the package to have the following information in English:
      a. The name and business address of the manufacturer, packer, distributor, or seller;
      b. The common or usual or chemical name of each hazardous ingredient;
      c. The signal word "Danger" for products that are corrosive, extremely flammable, or highly toxic;
      d. The signal word "Caution" or "Warning" for all other hazardous products;
      e. An affirmative statement of the principal hazard or hazards that the product presents (e.g., "Flammable," "Harmful if Swallowed," "Causes Burns," "Vapor Harmful," etc.);
      f. Precautionary statements telling users what they must do or what actions they must avoid to protect themselves;
      g. Where it is appropriate, instructions for first aid treatment if the product injures someone;

      h. The word "Poison" for a product that is highly toxic, in addition to the signal word "Danger";
      i. If a product requires special care in handling or storage, instructions for consumers to follow to protect themselves; and
      j. The statement "Keep out of the reach of children." If a hazardous product such as a plant does not have a package, it still must have a hang tag that contains the required precautionary information. That information must also be printed in any literature that accompanies the product and that contains instructions for use.
  3. The act does not apply to drugs regulated by FDA, but may apply to other products sold in a pharmacy such as bleach, cleaning fluids, antifreeze, etc.

B. Hazard Communication Standard
  1. The Occupational and Safety Health Administration (OSHA) administers and enforces this regulation, which requires employers (including pharmacies) that deal with hazardous materials to meet the Hazard Communication Standard. *See 29 CFR 1910.1200*
  2. The standard requires chemical manufacturers and importers to classify the hazards of chemicals they produce or import and to prepare appropriate labels and Safety Data Sheets (SDS), which were formerly known as Material Safety Data Sheets (MSDS).
  3. Drugs in solid, final dosage form for administration to patients are exempt from these requirements, but hazardous chemicals or products not in solid, final dosage form for administration (such as liquid products used in compounding) may be covered. Generally, a pharmacy may rely on the manufacturer to determine if a product is considered hazardous. If a pharmacy has any such products, they are required to have a written Hazard Communication Plan.
  4. The plan must include a list of hazardous chemicals in the workplace, must ensure all such products are appropriately labeled and have a Safety Data Sheet, and must include training for all workers on the hazards of chemicals, appropriate protective measures, and where and how to obtain additional information.

Note: Additional details can be found in OSHA's publication "Small Entity Compliance Guide for Employers that Use Hazardous Chemicals."

C. Centers for Medicare and Medicaid Services (CMS) Requirements
  1. Tamper-Resistant Prescriptions—CMS requires that all written prescriptions meet certain tamper-resistant requirements to prevent unauthorized copying and to prevent counterfeiting (with some exceptions). The tamper-evident features must include:
     a. One or more industry-recognized features designed to prevent unauthorized copying of a completed or blank prescription form;
     b. One or more industry-recognized features designed to prevent the erasure or modification of information written on the prescription pad by the prescriber; and
     c. One or more industry-recognized features designed to prevent the use of counterfeit prescription forms.
  2. Pharmacy Services at Long Term Care Facilities:
     a. Medication Regimen Reviews—CMS regulations require a consultant pharmacist to perform a Medication Regimen Review for all long-term care patients every 30 days. The pharmacist must report any irregularities to the attending physician, the facility's medical director, and the facility's director of nursing, and these reports must be acted upon.
     b. PRN orders for psychotropic drugs must be limited to 14 days unless the practitioner documents the rationale for extending an order beyond 14 days. PRN orders for psychotropic drugs cannot be renewed unless the attending physician evaluates the resident for appropriateness of that drug.

D. Delivering Prescriptions by U.S. Mail or Common Carrier
  1. Delivery by Mail (postal regulations administered by the U.S. Postal Service)—General postal regulations do not allow dangerous substances to be mailed; however, there are exceptions for prescription drugs.
     a. Non-controlled—Prescriptions containing non-controlled substances may be mailed by a pharmacy to the ultimate user provided that the medications are not alcoholic beverages, poisons, or flammable substances.

        b. Controlled substances may be mailed to patients under the following requirements:
- **(1)** The prescription container must be labeled in compliance with prescription labeling rules;
- **(2)** The outer wrapper or container in which the prescription is placed must be free of markings that would indicate the nature of the contents (including the name of the pharmacy as part of the return address on the mailing package, as that may alert individuals that drugs may be in the package); and
- **(3)** No markings of any kind may be placed on the package to indicate the nature of contents.

        c. Controlled substances may be mailed to other DEA registrants (practitioners, other pharmacies, distributors, or drug disposal firms) provided they are placed in a plain outer container or securely overwrapped in plain paper and all recordkeeping requirements are met.

    2. Delivery by Common Carrier—Any prescription drug may be delivered from a pharmacy to a patient by common carrier such as the United Parcel Service (UPS) or FedEx. This includes all schedules of controlled substances and dangerous drugs. Common carriers are not subject to postal regulations.

E. Federal Tax-Free Alcohol Regulations
1. Pharmacies sometimes use 95% ethanol (190 proof) for compounding purposes.
2. When used for scientific, medicinal, or mechanical purposes or to treat patients, such alcohol is considered "tax free."
3. The Alcohol and Tobacco Tax and Trade Bureau (TTB) regulates tax-free alcohol with the federal Bureau of Alcohol, Tobacco, Firearms, and Explosives (ATFE). ATFE is responsible for enforcement.
4. A user permit must be acquired from TTB and specific recordkeeping requirements must be met.
5. Tax-free alcohol cannot be resold or used in any beverage product.

VI. Privacy—HIPAA and HITECH (Enforced by the Office of Civil Rights)
A. Most pharmacies are a "covered entity" under HIPAA and must be in compliance with these requirements.

B. Notice and Acknowledgement
1. Pharmacies must provide patients with a "Notice of Privacy Practices" and make a good faith effort to obtain a written acknowledgement of receipt of the Notice from the patient.
2. The Notice must be provided upon first service delivery to the patient.
3. The HIPAA privacy rule requires mandatory provisions in the Notice.

C. Use and Disclosure of Protected Health Information (PHI)
1. Protected Health Information (PHI) is the HIPAA term for patient-identifiable information.
2. Pharmacies may use and disclose PHI to provide treatment for payment and for healthcare operations without authorization from the patient.
3. Pharmacies may also use and disclose PHI for certain governmental functions without authorization from the patient. This includes uses and disclosures for public health activities such as reporting adverse events to FDA, to health oversight agencies such as boards of pharmacies or state drug monitoring programs, and to law enforcement agencies.
4. Other uses and disclosures, such as for marketing purposes, require a signed authorization from the patient. If the covered entity receives remuneration for the marketing, the authorization form must expressly inform the patient of such.
5. Face-to-face communications about alternative drugs or health products are considered part of treatment and not marketing.
6. Refill reminders for a currently prescribed drug (or one that has lapsed for not more than 90 days) are not considered marketing as long as any payment made to the pharmacy in exchange for making the communication is reasonable and related to the pharmacy's cost of making the communication.
7. Minimum Necessary Standard
    a. When using and disclosing PHI, a pharmacy must make reasonable efforts to limit PHI to the minimum necessary to accomplish the intended purpose.
    b. The minimum necessary standard does not apply to disclosures to healthcare providers for treatment purposes.

These disclosures would include prescription transfers or providing prescription information to physicians.
- c. The minimum necessary standard does not apply to disclosures for which the patient has signed an authorization.
- d. The minimum necessary standard does apply to disclosures for payment.
8. Incidental Disclosures
- a. Unintended "incidental" disclosures are not a violation of the Privacy Rule as long as reasonable safeguards are in place.
- b. Examples: Sales representatives or janitorial service members accidentally see PHI during the normal course of their jobs; a customer overhears counseling that is performed in a private area in a discreet manner.

D. Business Associates (BAs)
1. BAs are persons or entities, other than members of a pharmacy's workforce, who perform a function or service on behalf of the pharmacy that requires the use or disclosure of PHI.
2. Pharmacies are required to enter into business associate contracts with these BAs, which require the BAs to meet many of the same requirements for protecting PHI as a covered entity under HIPAA.

E. Patient Rights and Administrative Requirements
1. Patients have a right to access and obtain a copy of their PHI. Pharmacies must comply with a request within 30 days, but may extend time by no more than 30 additional days if they notify the individual of the reason for the delay.
2. Patients have a right to amend their PHI records and request an accounting of disclosures of their PHI made by a pharmacy under certain circumstances. Pharmacies must comply with a request to amend or request for an accounting of disclosures within 60 days, but may extend it by no more than 30 additional days if they notify the individual of the reason for the delay.
3. Pharmacies must establish policies and procedures to protect from accidental or intentional uses and disclosures of PHI through the use of appropriate administrative, technical, and physical safeguards to protect the privacy of PHI.

4. Pharmacies must train all employees on privacy policies and impose sanctions on employees for any violations of privacy policies.
5. Pharmacies must designate a Privacy Official who is responsible for development and implementation of HIPAA-related policies, procedures, and compliance.
6. Pharmacies must also designate a contact person to receive complaints. This person may also be the Privacy Official.

F. HITECH Act—The HITECH Act amended HIPAA to strengthen many of its provisions. Among other things, the HITECH Act added a breach notification requirement that requires:
1. Covered Entities, including pharmacies, to notify individuals of a breach of their "unsecured" PHI within 60 calendar days after the breach is discovered.
2. BAs must report any breaches of unsecured PHI to the covered entity and provide the identities of each affected individual.
3. A "breach" is defined as unauthorized acquisition, access, use, or disclosure of PHI that compromises its security or privacy. It does not include instances in which there has been an inadvertent disclosure from an authorized individual to another person authorized to access PHI within the same organization. A breach also does not include instances in which the covered entity or BA has a good faith belief that the PHI is not further acquired, accessed, retained, used, or disclosed.
4. For breaches affecting fewer than 500 individuals, covered entities must maintain a log of these breaches and notify HHS of these breaches annually.
5. If more than 500 individuals are affected, the Secretary of HHS and prominent local media must be notified in addition to the affected individuals within 60 days after the breach is discovered.

CHAPTER TWO
Federal Controlled Substances Act (FCSA) and Florida Controlled Substances Act (FLCSA) and Applicable Rules

CHAPTER TWO
Federal Controlled Substances Act (FCSA) and Florida Controlled Substances Act (FLCSA) and Applicable Rules

Note: Throughout this chapter, unless otherwise noted, requirements listed as part of the FCSA are the same under the FLCSA.

I. **Drug Classification**
   A. Schedule I (C-I) Drugs
      1. High potential for abuse and severe potential for dependence (addiction).
      2. No currently accepted medical use in treatment in the U.S.
      3. Lack of accepted information on the safety of their use under medical supervision.
      4. Include opiates and derivatives such as heroin and dihydromorphine; hallucinogens such as marijuana, lysergic acid diethylamide (LSD), peyote, and mescaline; and depressants such as methaqualone.

STUDY TIP: While Florida and many other states have "legalized" the medical or recreational use of marijuana, it is still a Schedule I controlled substance under federal law and is technically illegal. Since the stricter law applies, for purposes of the MPJE it is recommended that you treat marijuana as a Schedule I controlled substance.

   B. Schedule II (C-II) Drugs
      1. High potential for abuse.
      2. Have currently accepted medical use in treatment in the U.S. or currently accepted medical use with severe restrictions.
      3. Abuse of the drug or other substances may lead to severe physical or psychological dependence (addiction).
      4. Include opium and other narcotics such as morphine, codeine, dihydrocodeine, oxycodone, acetaminophen with hydrocodone (Vicodin®), methadone, meperidine, hydromorphone, fentanyl, and cocaine; stimulants such as amphetamine, methamphetamine, phenmetrazine, and methylphenidate; and depressants such as pentobarbital, secobarbital, amobarbital, glutethimide, and phencyclidine.

STUDY TIP: The term "narcotic" refers to drugs that are derivatives of opium, poppy straw, cocaine, or ecgonine. While all narcotics are controlled substances, not all controlled substances are narcotics.

C. Schedule III (C-III) Drugs
   1. Potential for abuse less than Schedule I or II.
   2. Have currently accepted medical use in treatment in the U.S.
   3. Abuse of the drug or other substance may lead to moderate or low physical dependence (addiction) or high psychological dependence (addiction).
   4. Include some narcotic Schedule II drugs, but in combination with another ingredient such as aspirin with codeine or acetaminophen with codeine (e.g., Tylenol #3). Also include some non-narcotic drugs, including suppository forms of amobarbital, secobarbital, or pentobarbital; stimulants such as chlorphentermine, phendimetrazine, and benzphetamine; anabolic steroids including testosterone; ketamine; paregoric; and Fiorinal®, a combination of butalbital, aspirin, and caffeine.

   Note: While Fiorinal® is a Schedule III controlled substance, Fioricet®, a combination of butalbital, acetaminophen, and caffeine, is an exempt prescription drug product (see D. below) and is not labeled as a controlled substance under federal law. Some states do schedule Fioricet® as a controlled substance, but Florida does not.

STUDY TIP: Under federal law, the suppository forms of amobarbital, secobarbital, and pentobarbital are Schedule III, but other dosage forms are Schedule II. The Florida Controlled Substances Act does not contain this distinction, however, and includes all dosage forms of these products under Schedule II.

D. Schedule IV (C-IV) Drugs
   1. Low potential for abuse relative to Schedule III.
   2. Have currently accepted medical use in treatment in the U.S.
   3. Abuse may lead to limited physical or psychological dependence (addiction) relative to Schedule III.
   4. Include narcotics such as dextropropoxyphene and products with not more than 1 mg of difenoxin and not less than 25 mcgs of atropine sulfate per dosage unit; depressants such as alprazolam, chloral hydrate, diazepam, lorazepam, and

phenobarbital; stimulants such as diethylpropion and phentermine; and other drugs such as carisoprodol, tramadol, pentazocine, and butorphanol.

STUDY TIP: Be careful with drugs that have similar names but are in different schedules, such as phenmetrazine (C-II), phendimetrazine (C-III), and phentermine (C-IV).

E. Schedule V (C-V) Drugs
   1. Low potential for abuse relative to Schedule IV.
   2. Have currently accepted medical use in treatment in the U.S.
   3. Abuse of the drug or other substance may lead to limited physical or psychological dependence (addiction) relative to Schedule IV.
   4. Include pregabalin (Lyrica®), antitussive products containing codeine, and antidiarrheal products containing opium.

STUDY TIP: The 2018 Farm Bill made hemp and hemp derivatives including cannabidiol (CBD) containing no more than 0.3% tetrahydrocannabinol (THC) non-controlled substances. However, FDA-approved cannabidiol derived from cannabis containing no more than 0.1% THC, such as Epidiolex®, were originally placed into Schedule V. In 2020, DEA removed these products from Schedule V, so they are no longer controlled substances under federal law. As of the date of publication of this book, Florida had not yet removed Epidiolex® from Schedule V, but was expected to do that to match the federal law.

F. Exempted Prescription Drug Products
   1. Manufacturers may apply to DEA to exempt a product or chemical from certain provisions of the Controlled Substances Act (labeling and inventory) if the product or chemical is not likely to be abused. These products may still be considered controlled substances for certain criminal violations even though they are not labeled as controlled substances.
   2. Exempted prescription drug preparations include non-narcotic products containing small amounts of phenobarbital, butalbital, chlordiazepoxide, or meprobamate. A common example is Fioricet® (butalbital, acetaminophen, and caffeine).
   3. The DEA Exempt Prescription Product List can be found on DEA's website.

- **G.** Listed Chemicals
  1. Listed Chemicals are chemicals that, in addition to legitimate uses, are used in manufacturing a controlled substance.
  2. In addition to specific chemicals, OTC products containing ephedrine, pseudoephedrine, or phenylpropanolamine are considered Listed Chemicals.
  Note: Ephedrine and phenylpropanolamine products have been removed from the market by FDA for safety reasons.
  3. These products are not controlled substance under federal law but are subject to certain sales limitations and other restrictions. *See Section X.D. below.*
- **H.** Scheduling of Controlled Substances
  1. Federal—U.S. Attorney General, as head of the Department of Justice (which DEA is under), may add, delete, or reschedule substances but must obtain a scientific and medical recommendation from FDA.
  2. State—The Florida Attorney General may add, delete, or reschedule substances under the FLCSA.

II. Scheduling of Compounded Controlled Substances

- **A.** A pharmacy may compound narcotic controlled substances pursuant to a prescription as long as the concentration is not greater than 20%. This 20% concentration limit applies to aqueous or oleaginous solutions or solid oral dosage forms. *See chart of coincident activities allowed at 21 CFR 1301.13.* DEA may consider compounding a narcotic prescription greater than 20% to be manufacturing, which would require the pharmacy to be registered with DEA as a manufacturer.
- **B.** The narcotic substance must be compounded with one or more non-narcotic therapeutic ingredients.

STUDY TIP: You should know the concentration limits for codeine and opium products and be able to calculate what schedule a particular compounded product would fall into. However, first be sure that the codeine or opium is being compounded with another non-narcotic therapeutic agent. Any prescription for a narcotic that is not mixed with another drug, regardless of concentration, will always be in Schedule II. For example, if codeine or opium is only being mixed with water or simple syrup, it is still a Schedule II, regardless of the concentration.

- **C.** Concentration limits
  1. Codeine
     a. C-V limit = 200 mg/100 ml.
     b. C-III limit = 1.8 g/100 ml and 90 mg/dosage unit. *Note: Anything above this limit would be Schedule II.*

STUDY TIP: Products such as Cheracol® and Robitussin AC® contain the maximum amount of codeine allowed for Schedule V. If you add any amount of codeine to these products, they would then be Schedule III.

  2. Opium
     a. C-V limit = 100 mg/100 ml.
     b. C-III limit (Federal law) = 500 mg/100 ml and 25 mg/dosage unit.
     c. C-III limit (Florida law)—None listed.
        Note: It is difficult to say if this was done intentionally or is simply an oversight in the Florida law, but the Florida controlled substance schedules do not have the federal Schedule III limit of 500 mg/100 ml for opium products compounded with another pharmaceutical ingredient. The Florida law does contain a limit for opium for Schedule V of 100mg/100ml. This means that under Florida law, any compounded opium product greater than 100mg/100ml goes from Schedule V straight to Schedule II.

STUDY TIP: A compounded narcotic prescription will never be a Schedule IV.

III. Registration
- **A.** General Information
  1. Every person or firm that manufactures, distributes, or dispenses any controlled substances or proposes to engage in any of these activities must register with DEA.
  2. There is no state controlled substance registration in Florida.
  3. Dispensers (pharmacies and practitioners) register every 3 years with DEA.
  4. Registration form for dispensers, including pharmacies, is DEA Form 224. Renewal form for dispensers is DEA Form 224a.
  5. Registration for dispensers is valid for 3 years.
  6. Dispenser registrations start with the letters "A," "B," or "F" (or "G" for Department of Defense contractors).

7. The second letter of the prefix will normally be the first letter of the practitioner's last name for individual practitioners or the first letter of a pharmacy's or hospital's name.

B. Mid-Level Practitioners
1. Registration begins with the letter "M."
2. May include advanced practice registered nurses and physician assistants if the state allows them to prescribe controlled substances. Other mid-level practitioners may include ambulance services, animal shelters, and veterinary euthanasia technicians.

C. Activities Requiring Separate Registrations
1. Manufacturing (C-I–C-V)
2. Distributing (C-I–C-V)
3. Reverse Distributing (C-I–C-V)
4. Dispensing (C-II–C-V)—Includes prescribing and administration by practitioners and dispensing by pharmacies
5. Conducting research (C-I)
6. Conducting research (C-II–C-V)
7. Conducting narcotic treatment program (C-II–C-V)
8. Conducting chemical analysis (C-I–C-V)
9. Importing (C-I–C-V)
10. Exporting (C-I–C-V)

Note: On October 5, 2020, DEA issued a notice of proposed rulemaking that includes a new category of registration for an Emergency Medical Services Agency. At the time of publication of this book, this proposed rule had not been finalized.

D. Verifying a DEA Registration (number)
1. Step 1—Add 1st, 3rd, and 5th digits.
2. Step 2—Add 2nd, 4th, and 6th digits and multiply sum by 2.
3. Step 3—Add the sum of steps 1 and 2, and the last digit of the sum should correspond to the last digit of the DEA number.
4. Example: DEA # AB1234563.
   a. $1 + 3 + 5 = 9$.
   b. $(2 + 4 + 6) \times 2 = 24$.
   c. Total = 33.

E. Separate registration is required for separate locations.
1. Each pharmacy must have a separate DEA registration.
2. DEA will sometimes issue a campus registration that may include multiple buildings for large hospitals or healthcare facilities, but this is done on a case-by-case basis.

3. Individual practitioners, including physicians who register at one location but practice at other locations in the same state, are not required to register at those other locations if they only prescribe controlled substances at those other locations. If a practitioner maintains a supply of controlled substances at a second site or if the second site is in another state, he or she would have to have an additional DEA registration for that site.

F. Application for Registration
1. DEA Form 224 for dispensers (practitioners and pharmacies).
2. Application must be signed (or electronically signed) by the applicant if for an individual, by a partner if it is for a partnership, or by an officer if it is for a corporation.
3. An applicant can authorize another individual to sign the application and renewals by filling out a Power of Attorney granting that individual the authority and filing that Power of Attorney with the DEA Registration Unit.

Note: This may be needed if a company (a hospital corporation or a pharmacy corporation) wishes to have a pharmacist be responsible for applying and renewing the DEA registration but the pharmacist is not an officer of the corporation. Unlike the Power of Attorney to sign DEA Form 222, this Power of Attorney must be filed with DEA. See Section IV. A.7. below.

G. Exemptions (i.e., who does not have to register with DEA)
1. An agent or employee of any registered manufacturer, distributor, or dispenser if acting in the usual course of business or employment.

STUDY TIP: Exempted persons would include pharmacists working in a pharmacy and nurses working in a hospital or physician's office.

2. A common or contract carrier or warehouseman or an employee thereof whose possession is in the usual course of business or employment.
3. An ultimate user (patient) who possesses such substance for a lawful purpose.
4. Officials of the U.S. Armed Services, Public Health Service, or Bureau of Prisons acting in the course of their official duties.

> *Note: Military and federal practitioners are exempt from having to register with DEA, and a pharmacy outside of the federal facility may legally fill a prescription issued by such a practitioner. In practice, this is difficult because many pharmacy computer systems will not allow a controlled substance to be filled without a valid prescriber's DEA number, and reporting to prescription monitoring programs may not work without a DEA number. For this reason, many federal practitioners choose to obtain a DEA registration.*

H. Practitioner's Use of Hospital DEA Number
   1. Interns, residents, staff physicians, and mid-level practitioners who are agents or employees of a hospital or other institution may administer, dispense, or prescribe controlled substances under the registration of the hospital or other institution when acting in the usual course of business or employment.
   2. The hospital must assign a specific internal code for each practitioner authorized to use the hospital's DEA number, and this must be available at all times to other registrants and law enforcement agencies. This internal code shall be a suffix to the hospital's DEA number (e.g., AP1234563-10 or AP1234563-A12).
   3. Controlled substance prescriptions written by these practitioners are valid and can be filled by any pharmacy, not just the hospital pharmacy where they are employed.

I. Temporary Use of Registration Upon Sale of a Pharmacy
   When selling a pharmacy, if the new owner has not yet obtained a DEA registration, DEA permits the new owner to continue the business of the pharmacy under the previous owner's registration, provided the following requirements are met:
   1. The new owner must expeditiously apply for an appropriate DEA registration and state licensure.
   2. The previous owner grants a Power of Attorney to the new owner that provides for the following:
      a. The previous owner agrees to allow the controlled substance activities of the pharmacy to be carried out under his or her DEA registration;
      b. The previous owner agrees to allow the new owner to carry out the controlled substance activities of the pharmacy, including the ordering of controlled substances, as an agent of the previous owner;

    c. The previous owner acknowledges, as the registrant, that he or she will be held accountable for any violations of controlled substance laws that may occur; and

    d. The previous owner agrees that the controlled substance activities of the pharmacy may be carried out under his or her DEA registration and shall remain in effect for no more than 45 days after the purchase date.

STUDY TIP: This temporary use procedure is not in a DEA rule. It was authorized many years ago in a policy letter from DEA. It is a practical policy to allow the new owner time to obtain a DEA registration after a change in ownership while still allowing patients to obtain refills and get prescriptions filled. An owner cannot apply for a DEA registration until they have their state pharmacy license and state controlled substance license if applicable. The 45-day limitation was in the original guidance from DEA, but some local DEA offices may permit a longer time period if needed.

IV. Ordering and Transferring Controlled Substances
  A. Ordering Schedule II Controlled Substances—DEA Form 222
    1. Required for each sale or transfer of C-II drugs (except dispensing to ultimate user).
    2. Only one item may be ordered on each numbered line.
    3. Orders for etorphine hydrochloride and diprenorphine must contain only orders for these substances.
    4. The number of lines completed must be noted on the form.
    5. Name and address of supplier from whom the controlled substances are being ordered must be entered.
    6. Must be signed (or electronically signed) by the registrant (individual, partner, or officer) or by the person authorized to execute DEA Form 222. *See 7. below.*
    7. Registrant may authorize other individuals to execute forms by creating a Power of Attorney (POA). This Power of Attorney does not need to be sent to DEA but must be maintained in the pharmacy. A POA must be signed by the person granting the power, the person receiving the power (called the attorney-in-fact), and two witnesses. A sample DEA Power of Attorney can be found in the DEA's Pharmacist Manual and at 21 CFR 1305.05(c).

STUDY TIP: Previously, DEA allowed the person who signed the last application or renewal to issue a POA to allow other individuals to sign DEA Form 222. Remember, that person may have signed the renewal application based on a POA from the registrant. That provision was removed effective October 30, 2019. This means that only the actual registrant may grant a POA for signing DEA Form 222.

8. Forms that are not complete, legible, properly prepared, or signed will not be accepted.
9. Forms that show any alteration, erasure, or changes will not be accepted.
10. A supplier may provide a partial quantity for the requested amount, but the remaining quantity must be sent within 60 days or the order becomes void. With the exception of certain Department of Defense orders, no DEA Form 222 is valid more than 60 days after its execution by the purchaser.
11. If a completed order form is lost or stolen, purchaser must prepare another DEA Form 222 along with a statement containing the serial number and date of the lost form and stating that the goods covered by the first order were not received because the form was lost.
12. A pharmacy may fax a completed DEA Form 222 to a supplier in order for the supplier to prepare the order; however, the supplier may not ship the product until the original DEA Form 222 is received and verified.
13. Single Copy DEA Form 222
    a. Effective October 30, 2019, DEA finalized new rules to transition from a triplicate (3 copy) DEA Form 222 to a single copy DEA Form 222 with additional security features. There is a 2-year transition period during which existing triplicate DEA Forms 222 can continue to be used.
    b. The new single forms contain 20 order lines per form rather than 10 order lines on the triplicate forms.
    c. The purchaser filling out a single copy DEA Form 222 must make a copy of the original form for its records and submit the original form to the supplier. The copy may be retained in paper or electronic form.
    d. The supplier may only fill an order from the original form and not from a copy. The supplier must record on

the original form its DEA registration number, the number of containers furnished for each ordered item, and the date the products are shipped to the purchaser.
   e. Most suppliers (e.g., wholesalers) are required to report the acquisition and disposition of Schedule II and certain Schedule III and IV controlled substances to DEA's Automation of Reports and Consolidated Orders System (ARCOS). A supplier who reports transactions to ARCOS is not required to send a copy of the original DEA Form 222 to DEA because this information is already reported to ARCOS. However, if a supplier is not required to report transactions to ARCOS (e.g., a pharmacy or practitioner acting as a supplier under the 5% rule), they must submit a copy of the original DEA Form 222 to DEA either by mail or by email to DEA.Orderforms@usdoj.gov when acting as a supplier.
   f. When the product has been received, the purchaser must record the number of containers received and the date received for each item on the copy of the DEA Form 222 they made when ordering the product.
   g. Registrants may continue to use existing triplicate DEA Forms 222 using the procedures outlined below until October 30, 2021.
14. Triplicate DEA Form 222
   a. Existing triplicate DEA Forms 222 may continue to be used until October 30, 2021.
   b. Triplicate DEA Forms 222 contain 10 order lines per form.
   c. Purchaser fills out the name and address of the supplier, date ordered, and products ordered. Only one product per line may be ordered, although multiple packages of each product can be ordered.
   d. The total number of lines ordered must be filled out and the form must be signed.
   e. Copies 1 (brown) and 2 (green) go to the supplier and may not be separated.
   f. Purchaser retains copy 3 (blue) for their records.
   g. Supplier indicates the number of packages shipped and date shipped on each line, sends copy 2 to the DEA, and retains copy 1 for their records.

    h. Upon receipt of the product, the purchaser records on the retained copy 3 the number of packages received and the date received for each line.
    i. Once the order is complete, copy 3 should be filed separately or attached to any Schedule II invoices that were received. *Note: The official record of receipt of a Schedule II controlled substance is copy 3 of the triplicate DEA Form 222 or the copy made by the purchaser of the single DEA Form 222 on which the quantity received and date is recorded, but many suppliers also send an invoice.*

STUDY TIP: It is important to understand how each copy of DEA Form 222 is handled, including where each copy is sent or kept. Normally the pharmacy is the purchaser, but in cases where the pharmacy is sending controlled substances to another DEA registrant (such as another pharmacy, a physician, or a reverse distributor), the pharmacy would be acting as the supplier. The purchaser always provides DEA Form 222 to the supplier.

15. Electronic Ordering of Schedule II Controlled Substances
    a. DEA allows electronic ordering of Schedule II controlled substances through the Controlled Substances Ordering System (CSOS).
    b. Each pharmacy must appoint a CSOS coordinator, who will serve as that pharmacy's recognized agent, regarding issues pertaining to issuance of, revocation of, and changes to digital certificates issued under that registrant's DEA registration.
    c. It allows electronic orders based on digital certificates issued by the DEA Certification Authority that are valid until the expiration of the DEA registration for the facility (3 years).
    d. Even though each CSOS Certificate expires when the DEA registration of the facility expires, they are issued to individual subscribers. Certificates must never be used by anyone other than the individual subscriber (a person, not a location) the certificate was issued to.
    e. There are two types of CSOS Certificates:
        (1) CSOS Administrative Certificates are used to digitally sign communications with DEA as well as with other participants in the CSOS community.

Administrative Certificates are issued only to CSOS Coordinators and are not valid for electronic ordering.

(2) CSOS Signing Certificates are used for digitally signing controlled substance orders. Signing certificates are issued to approved Registrant and Power of Attorney applicants. Approved Coordinator applicants will only be issued a Signing certificate if he/she holds valid Power of Attorney for controlled substance ordering and has requested a Signing certificate on his/her CSOS Certificate Application.

f. All CSOS applications must be audited by an independent third-party auditor prior to use and whenever changes are made to the software to ensure that the software is in compliance with DEA regulations.

g. An electronic order for controlled substances may not be filled if any of the following occurs:
  (1) The required data fields have not been completed.
  (2) The order is not signed using a digital certificate issued by DEA.
  (3) The digital certificate used has expired or been revoked prior to signature.
  (4) The purchaser's public key will not validate the digital certificate.
  (5) The validation of the order shows that the order is invalid for any reason.

h. If an order cannot be filled, the supplier must notify the purchaser and provide a statement as to the reason (e.g., improperly prepared or altered). A supplier may, for any reason, refuse to accept any order. If a supplier refuses, a statement that the order is not accepted is sufficient.

i. When a purchaser receives an unaccepted electronic order from the supplier, the purchaser must electronically link the statement of nonacceptance to the original order. The original statement must be retained for two years. Neither a purchaser nor a supplier may correct a defective order. The purchaser must issue a new order for the order to be filled.

Note: For details on CSOS, see DEA's eCommerce website at https://www.deaecom.gov/csosmain.html.

B. Ordering Schedule III–V Controlled Substances
  1. Schedule III–V controlled substances can be ordered through normal ordering processes from a wholesaler or manufacturer, but must be documented by a pharmacy with an invoice provided by the wholesaler or manufacturer.
  2. The invoice must contain:
     a. Name of controlled substance.
     b. Dosage form and strength.
     c. Number of units per container (e.g., 100-tablet bottle).
     d. Quantity received (containers).
     e. Date of receipt.
     f. Name, address, and DEA number of the registrant from where the controlled substance was received.

STUDY TIP: It is recommended that you memorize the required elements on an invoice for controlled substances.

C. Transfers of Controlled Substances—The 5% Rule
  1. A pharmacy does not have to register with DEA as a distributor as long as total quantities of controlled substances distributed during a 12-month period in which the pharmacy is registered do not exceed 5% of the total quantity of all controlled substances dispensed and distributed during that same 12-month period.
  2. Example: A pharmacy dispenses and distributes a total of 10,000 doses (i.e., tablets, capsules, teaspoons, etc.) of all controlled substances (not just C-II drugs). This pharmacy would be allowed to transfer 500 doses without being registered with DEA as a distributor.
  3. If the transfer is for a Schedule II controlled substance, a DEA Form 222 is required. For Schedule III–V controlled substances, an invoice provided by the supplier (i.e., the pharmacy) is required with all of the required elements as listed in B.2. above.
  4. Transfers can only be made to the address listed on a DEA registration. This applies to all controlled substances, not just Schedule II controlled substances.

STUDY TIP: Notice that for Schedule II controlled substances, the person receiving the product initiates and fills out the DEA Form 222, which is sent to the supplier or seller. However, for Schedule III–V controlled substances, the invoice is provided by the supplier or seller to the purchaser.

V. Additional Requirements for Controlled Substances
A. Storage and Security
1. Pharmacies may store controlled substances in a secure cabinet that is locked.
2. Pharmacies may store controlled substances by dispersal throughout the non-controlled stock to deter theft.
3. Pharmacies may not store all controlled substances on one unsecured shelf.

STUDY TIP: While many pharmacies keep some or all of their controlled substances in locked storage, it is not a legal requirement.

B. Theft or Significant Loss
1. A theft or significant loss of controlled substances must be reported in writing to DEA within one business day of discovery of the theft or significant loss. DEA also recommends notifying local police.

STUDY TIP: Any theft must be reported, but only "significant" losses.

2. Florida law also requires notification of a theft or significant loss of controlled substances to the county sheriff within 24 hours upon discovery. Failure to do so is a first degree misdemeanor. *See FLCSA § 893.07(5)(b)*
3. FPA § 465.022(11)(b) requires the prescription department manager (PDM) of a pharmacy to notify the Florida Board of Pharmacy of any theft or significant loss of any controlled substances within one business day after discovery of the theft or loss. *Note: The language in the statute says this is a requirement of the prescription department manager, but institutional pharmacies do not have a prescription department manager. They have a consultant pharmacist of record (see Chapter 3). Despite the language in the statute, it is likely that the intent of this law is that this reporting requirement also applies to a consultant pharmacist of record for an institutional pharmacy.*

4. Complete DEA Form 106 (Theft or Loss of Controlled Substances). This form can be filled out online at DEA's website.
5. Submitting DEA Form 106 immediately is not necessary if the pharmacy needs time to investigate the facts, but an initial notification must be provided in writing to DEA within one business day of discovery. If the investigation lasts longer than two months, the pharmacy needs to provide an update to DEA.
Note: At the time of publication of this book, DEA had proposed revising this rule to require that the DEA Form 106 be filed within 15 days of discovery. It also would require the form to be filled out online, which almost everyone already does. You should check to see if this rule was adopted as proposed or modified, although it is unlikely to be on the MPJE if it was only recently adopted.

C. Reporting Losses of Listed Chemicals (primarily pseudoephedrine products in a pharmacy)
1. DEA requires any unusual or excessive loss or disappearance (this would include a theft) of a listed chemical to be reported to DEA at the earliest practicable opportunity.
2. A written report must be provided within 15 days and must include a description of the circumstances of the loss (in-transit, theft from premises, etc.).

D. Miscellaneous DEA Rules and Policies
1. Convicted Felon Rule—A pharmacy cannot employ someone who has access to controlled substances if the person has been convicted of a felony involving controlled substances unless a waiver is granted by DEA.
2. Employee Screening Procedures—DEA requires pharmacies to screen potential employees with specific questions regarding criminal history and use of controlled substances.
3. Employee Responsibility to Report Drug Diversion—Individual employees are required to report any diversion by other employees to a responsible security official of the employer.
4. Federal Transfer Warning (21 CFR 209.5)—The following warning is required to be on the label of Schedule II–IV controlled substances when dispensed to a patient: "Caution: Federal law prohibits the transfer of this drug to any person other than the patient for whom it was prescribed." The only

exception would be for a controlled substance dispensed in a "blinded" clinical study.

STUDY TIP: Federal law requires the transfer warning only for Schedule II–IV controlled substances (not Schedule V). However, Florida law requires it for all controlled substance prescriptions, including Schedule V products. See FLCSA § 893.04(1)(e)7. Pharmacies generally comply with this requirement by including this language in small print on every prescription label, but it is legally only required for controlled substances.

- **E.** Disposal and Destruction of Controlled Substance Inventory (drugs not yet dispensed)
    - **1.** On-site destruction of controlled substances in a pharmacy.
        - **a.** Must be done using DEA Form 41, which requires the name and NDC number of the drug and the strength, dosage form, package size, and quantity of the controlled substances destroyed. It also requires recording the method by which the drugs were destroyed and two signatures of employees who witnessed the destruction. *Note: DEA Form 41 is also used to document destruction of controlled substances that a pharmacy received as an authorized collector even though these drugs are not stock controlled substances because they are not part of the pharmacy's inventory. See Section F.2. below.*
        - **b.** Destruction of controlled substances must be done in compliance with all state and federal laws, and the method of destruction shall be sufficient to render all such controlled substances non-retrievable. Because this is difficult to do, most community pharmacies do not use this method of destruction.
        - **c.** "Non-retrievable" is defined as "to permanently alter any controlled substance's physical and/or chemical condition or state through irreversible means in order to render the controlled substance unavailable and unusable for all practical purposes." *Note: This can be difficult to execute. In addition to the difficulty of complying with other laws such as EPA laws, DEA has stated that methods such as mixing controlled substances with items such as kitty litter or coffee grounds and depositing in the garbage do not meet the non-retrievable standard.*

       d. FBOP Rule 64B16-28.303 requires that pharmacies (other than Institutional Class I–nursing homes) using a DEA Form 41 for destruction to have the following sign the form as witnesses:

          (1) the prescription department manager or consultant pharmacist of record and a DEA agent or Department of Health inspector; or

          (2) the prescription department manager or consultant pharmacist of record and the medical director or his or her physician designee; or the director of nursing or his or her licensed nurse designee, or a sworn law enforcement officer.

STUDY TIP: The Florida rule on destruction using DEA Form 41 also states that the completed and witnessed DEA Form 41 must be sent to the closest DEA office within one business day of destruction. DEA's instructions on the DEA Form 41 state that the form is not required to be sent to DEA unless requested, but many DEA offices still require it. Since the Florida law specifically states a copy of the completed DEA Form 41 must be sent to DEA, it would be best to answer any question regarding this based on the Florida law.

---

    2. Transfer to an Authorized (Registered) Reverse Distributor

       a. This is the preferred method of destruction of controlled substance inventory in a pharmacy and is simply a transfer from one DEA registrant (the pharmacy) to another (the reverse distributor).

       b. Because this is a transfer, a DEA Form 41 is not required. The transfer must be documented with an invoice for Schedule III–V controlled substances and a DEA Form 222 for Schedule II controlled substances.

STUDY TIP: Be sure to understand the difference between use of a DEA Form 41, which is used to destroy controlled substances on the premises of a pharmacy (even though this is not often done in community practice), and transferring controlled substances to a DEA-registered reverse distributor for destruction, which requires a DEA Form 222 or an invoice.

  F. Disposal of Dispensed Controlled Substances at Nursing Homes and Collected from Ultimate Users and Other Non-Registrants

    1. Destruction of Controlled Substances at an Institutional Class I (Nursing Home) Pharmacy (Rule 64B16-28.301)

a. Controlled substances may be destroyed with documentation showing the name, quantity, strength, and dosage form of the drug, the patient's name, the prescription number, and the name of the institution.
  b. Destruction must be witnessed by at least two of the following:
      (1) Consultant pharmacist;
      (2) Director of nursing;
      (3) Facility administrator;
      (4) A licensed physician, mid-level practitioner, nurse, or another pharmacist employed by or under contract with the facility; or
      (5) A sworn law enforcement officer.
  c. The consultant pharmacist must review all controlled substance destruction documentation monthly to ensure compliance.

STUDY TIP: Notice that a DEA Form 41 is not required for destruction by a Class I Institutional Pharmacy (nursing home) because these drugs have already been dispensed to the patients. They are accounted for in the dispensing records of the pharmacy servicing that nursing home.

2. Authorized Collectors and DEA Take-Back Events
   a. DEA rules allow pharmacies to modify their DEA registrations to serve as a collector of controlled substances from ultimate users, including patients, the personal representative of the patient in the event of the patient's death, and at long-term care facilities (i.e., dispensed controlled substances).
   b. A pharmacy or hospital is not required to serve as a collector.
   c. The following rules apply to Authorized Collectors:
       (1) Collectors may allow ultimate users (patients) to deposit controlled substances into collection receptacles at the registered location or at an authorized long-term care facility (LTCF).
       (2) The controlled substances may be commingled with non-controlled substances.
       (3) The deposited substances may not be counted, sorted, inventoried, or individually handled. This means that the pharmacist should not be handling

these controlled substances on the patient's behalf. Patients must be the ones who place the controlled substances into the collection receptacles.

(4) LTCF staff may dispose of a patient's controlled substances into an authorized collection receptacle. Disposal into a collection receptacle must occur within three business days after the discontinuation of use by the patient.

(5) Collection receptacles must be in the immediate proximity (where they can be seen) of where controlled substances are stored (i.e., the pharmacy).

(6) Collection receptacles must be securely fastened to a permanent structure, locked, and securely constructed with a permanent outer container and a removable inner container.

(7) The inner liner must be waterproof, tamper-evident, removable, and able to be sealed immediately upon removal with no emptying or touching of the contents or ability to view the contents. The inner liner also must have a permanent unique identification number that allows tracking.

(8) The inner liner must be removed by or under the supervision of at least two employees of the Authorized Collector.

(9) Sealed inner liners may not be opened, x-rayed, analyzed, or otherwise penetrated.

(10) Collectors can either destroy the collected drugs on-site, transfer the collected drugs for final disposal to a DEA-registered reverse distributor, or contact the DEA Special Agent in Charge for assistance. If destroyed on-site, DEA Form 41 would be utilized. Section 2 of DEA Form 41 is for "collected substances." Instead of indicating the specific controlled substances being destroyed, it requires the unique identification number of the inner liner from the collection receptacle or the mail-back package.

d. A pharmacy that serves as a collector may also operate a mail-back program for collection of dispensed controlled substances. Packages used in a mail-back program must:

（1） Be nondescript and shall not have any markings or other information that might indicate that the package contains controlled substances;
（2） Be waterproof, tamper-evident, tear-resistant, and sealable;
（3） Be pre-addressed with and delivered to the collector's registered address;
（4） Include prepaid shipping costs;
（5） Have a unique identification number to enable tracking; and
（6） Include instructions for the user.

STUDY TIP: A collector that conducts a mail-back program may only accept packages that the collector made available. If the collector receives a package that it did not make available, the collector must notify DEA within three business days of receipt.

      e. DEA also conducts Drug Take Back Days to collect controlled substances (and other drugs) from ultimate users.
  3. Disposal of Controlled Substances of a Hospice Patient by Employees of the Hospice
      a. The SUPPORT Act, a comprehensive opioid bill passed by Congress in late 2018, authorizes an employee of a qualified hospice program to handle controlled substances, which were lawfully dispensed to a person receiving hospice care, for the purpose of destruction.
      b. DEA has yet to adopt regulations to implement this law.

G. Inventories
  1. An initial inventory is required on the first day the pharmacy is open for business.
  2. Both federal and Florida law require a controlled substance inventory biennially (every 2 years) and that inventory must be maintained in the pharmacy. The inventory may be done on the pharmacy's regular physical inventory date, which is nearest to, and does not vary by more than six months from, the biennial date that would apply.
  3. Newly scheduled drugs or drugs moved from one schedule to another must be inventoried on the day scheduled or moved to a new schedule.

4. Inventory Counts
   a. An exact count is required for all Schedule IIs.
   b. An estimated count is allowed for Schedule III–V products unless the container holds more than 1,000 tablets or capsules.

STUDY TIP: Although many pharmacies maintain a perpetual inventory of Schedule II controlled substances or even for all controlled substances, a perpetual inventory is not legally required.

H. Records
   1. Records of controlled substances must be maintained for 2 years under both the federal and Florida controlled substances acts.

STUDY TIP: Although federal and state law are consistent on this, there are certain records that may be required to be kept longer under other laws or rules, and these can sometimes include controlled substance records. For instance, Florida rules require that original prescription records be kept four years from the date of last dispensing, and that would include controlled substance prescriptions.

   2. DEA requires that records and inventories of Schedule II controlled substances be kept separately from all other records. Records and inventories of Schedule III–V controlled substances must be maintained separately or be "readily retrievable" from other records. "Readily retrievable" means the record is kept or maintained in such a manner that it can be separated out from all other records in a reasonable time or that it is identified by an asterisk, a redline, or some other identifiable manner such that it is easily distinguishable from all other records.
   3. Records of Receipt of Controlled Substances
      a. C-II—Copy 3 of DEA Form 222 or copy of original single page DEA Form 222 (with the number of containers and date received filled in).
      b. C-III–C-V—Supplier's invoice.
   4. Records of Disbursement of Controlled Substances
      a. Most pharmacies maintain records of dispensing in an electronic system (i.e., computer system). DEA has

specific requirements for electronic records of prescriptions as follows:
- **(1)** The electronic system must provide online retrieval of original prescription information and current refill history for those prescriptions which are currently authorized for refill.
- **(2)** The pharmacist must verify and document that the refill data entered into the system is correct.
- **(3)** The system must be able to produce a hard-copy printout of each day's controlled substance prescription refills, and each pharmacist who refilled those prescriptions must verify his/her accuracy by signing and dating the printout as he/she would sign a check or legal document. This daily printout must be printed within 72 hours of the date refills were dispensed. *Note: Most pharmacies do not print out this daily hard copy and instead use the alternative procedure in (4) below.*
- **(4)** Instead of the daily printout, a pharmacy can maintain a bound logbook or a separate file in which each pharmacist involved in the day's dispensing signs a statement verifying that the refill information entered into the computer that day has been reviewed by him/her and is correct as shown.
- **(5)** A pharmacy's electronic system must have the capability of printing out any refill data, which the pharmacy must maintain under the CSA. For example, this would include a refill-by-refill audit trail for any specified strength and dosage form of any controlled substance, by either brand or generic name or both, dispensed by the pharmacy. Such a printout must include:
   - **i.** Prescribing practitioner's name
   - **ii.** Patient's name and address
   - **iii.** Quantity and date dispensed on each refill
   - **iv.** Name or identification code of the dispensing pharmacist
   - **v.** Original prescription number.

b. Florida has a similar rule for electronic records of controlled substance prescriptions dispensed. *See Summary Record requirements in Section VI.A.4.(e.) below.*

STUDY TIP: These are antiquated rules, but you need to know them. These rules were put in place when pharmacies were transitioning from manual recordkeeping to electronic recordkeeping. In a manual recordkeeping system, DEA rules still require the pharmacist to document all refills of controlled substances on the back of the hard copy of the prescription by indicating the date refilled and the pharmacist's initials.

    c. Prescription files—Although most pharmacies maintain electronic dispensing records, there are still specific storage requirements for the hard copies of all written or verbal controlled substance prescriptions that were reduced to writing. Storage options:
       (1) 3-file storage system:
          File #1 = Schedule II only.
          File #2 = Schedule III–V.
          File #3 = Non-controlled drugs.
       (2) 2-file storage system:
          File #1—Schedule II only.
          File #2—Schedule III–V and non-controlled drugs. With this system, controlled substance prescriptions have to be stamped with red ink in the lower right corner of the prescription with a "C" (not less than 1 inch in height) so as to be readily retrievable from non-controlled substances.

Note: If a pharmacy maintains records in a data processing system for prescriptions (i.e., a computer) that permits identification by prescription number and retrieval of original documents by prescriber's name, patient's name, drug dispensed, and date filled, then the requirement to mark the hard-copy prescription with a red "C" is waived.

STUDY TIP: The file storage system requirements only apply to written prescriptions and verbal prescriptions that are reduced to writing by a pharmacist. If a controlled substance prescription is transmitted electronically, DEA requires that those electronic prescriptions be maintained electronically.

Other records of disbursement (i.e., controlled substances that leave a pharmacy) include DEA Form 106 (Theft or Significant Loss), DEA Form 41 (Destruction), DEA Form 222 for any Schedule II distributions made

under the 5% rule, and invoices for Schedule III–V distributions made under the 5% rule.
I. Central Recordkeeping
   1. A pharmacy wishing to maintain shipping and financial records at a central location other than the registered location must notify the nearest DEA Diversion Field Office.
   2. Unless the pharmacy is notified by DEA that permission to keep the central records is denied, the pharmacy may begin maintaining central records 14 days after notifying DEA.
   3. Central records shall not include executed (i.e., completed) DEA order forms (Copy 3 of DEA Form 222 or the copy made by the pharmacy of a single copy DEA Form 222), prescriptions, or inventories. These must be kept at the pharmacy.

STUDY TIP: Notice that unused DEA Form 222s may be kept at a central location, but once they have been executed (i.e., completed), they must be kept at the pharmacy. This is because the used DEA order form is the official record of the Schedule II controlled substances received. Be sure to know the records that cannot be kept at a central location.

VI. **Dispensing Controlled Substance Prescriptions**
   A. Corresponding Responsibility
      1. For a prescription for a controlled substance to be valid, it must be issued for a legitimate medical purpose by an individual practitioner acting in the usual scope of his or her professional practice.
      2. The responsibility for the proper prescribing and dispensing of a controlled substance is upon the prescribing practitioner, but a corresponding responsibility rests with the pharmacist who fills the prescription. This means a pharmacist cannot simply rely on the fact that a physician has a valid DEA registration to determine if a controlled substance prescription is valid.
      3. Through enforcement actions, DEA and the Florida Board of Pharmacy have identified a number of "red flags" that may require a pharmacist to do further investigation as to the legitimacy of controlled substance prescriptions.
      4. Standards of Practice for the Filling of Controlled Substance Prescriptions. *See FBOP Rule 64B16-27.831*
         a. General Standards for Validating a Prescription

STUDY TIP: This rule previously listed specific "red flags" that pharmacists should look for, but those specifics were later removed. Even though the specifics were removed, you should familiarize yourself with the most common red flags. Common red flags can be found in various sources online, including the NABP website.

      (1) Validating a prescription means the process implemented by the pharmacist to determine that the prescription was issued for a legitimate medical purpose.

      (2) If a pharmacist determines that, in his or her professional judgment, any concerns with the validity of the prescription cannot be resolved, the pharmacist shall refuse to fill or dispense the prescription.

  b. Minimum Standards Before Refusing to Fill a Prescription—Before refusing to fill a prescription based solely on concerns about the validity of the prescription, a pharmacist must attempt to:

      (1) Initiate communication with the patient to acquire relevant information;

      (2) Initiate communication with the prescriber to acquire relevant information;

      (3) In lieu of (1) or (2), but not both, the pharmacist may elect to access the PDMP to acquire relevant information.

Note: This rule was written prior to mandatory use of the PDMP and probably needs to be updated.

  c. Duty to Report—If a pharmacist has reason to believe that a prescriber is involved in the diversion of controlled substances, the pharmacist shall report such prescriber to the Florida Department of Health.

STUDY TIP: You should always take note of mandatory reporting requirements.

  d. Mandatory Continuing Education—The rule also requires a mandatory 2-hour continuing education on validation and counseling of prescriptions for Controlled Substances and Opioids, which must include:

      (1) Ensuring access to controlled substances for all patients with a valid prescription;

- (2) Use of the Prescription Drug Monitoring Program's Database;
- (3) Assessment of prescriptions for appropriate therapeutic value;
- (4) Detection of prescriptions not based on a legitimate medical purpose;
- (5) The laws and rules related to the prescribing and dispensing of controlled substances;
- (6) Proper patient storage and disposal of controlled substances;
- (7) Protocols for addressing and resolving problems recognized during the drug utilization review;
- (8) Education on the provision of Florida Statute § 381.887 on Emergency Treatment for Suspected Opioid Overdoses and on the State Surgeon General's Statewide Standing Order for Naloxone (eff. May 19, 2017) for as long as the Order is valid and effective;
- (9) Pharmacist-initiated counseling of patients with opioid prescriptions; and
- (10) Available treatment resources for opioid physical dependence, addiction, misuse, or abuse.

e. Summary Record
- (1) Every pharmacy must maintain a computerized record of controlled substances dispensed.
- (2) A hard-copy printout summary of such record covering the previous 60-day period shall be made available within 72 hours of request by any authorized law enforcement personnel.
- (3) The summary record must include information to be able to determine the volume (*Note: probably should say "quantity"*) and identity of controlled substances being dispensed under the prescription of a specific prescriber, and the volume (*Note: probably should say "quantity"*) and identity of controlled substances being dispensed to a specific patient.

Note: This is a curious requirement because all this information is reported to and is available in the PDMP. While law enforcement agencies do not have direct access to the PDMP, they may request information from the PDMP for an active investigation from the Department of Health if they have entered into a user agreement with the department. Since this language is still in the rule, pharmacies need to be able to provide this summary report from their computer within 72 hours upon request from authorized law enforcement personnel. Also note, a separate rule requires pharmacies to produce records of dispensing from the computer system for all prescriptions dispensed (not just controlled substances) upon request from an authorized agent of the Department of Health within 48 hours. See Rule 64B16-28.140

    5. Fraudulent Prescriptions—Duty to Report (§ 465.015(3))

        a. It is unlawful for any pharmacist to knowingly fail to report to the sheriff or other chief law enforcement agency of the county where the pharmacy is located of any instance that the pharmacist knew or believed a person obtained or attempted to obtain a controlled substance through fraudulent methods or representations.

        b. This report must be made within 24 hours after learning of the fraud or attempted fraud or at the close of the next business day, whichever is later.

B. Prescriptive Authority

    1. Who can prescribe controlled substance prescriptions is determined by state law. Florida law authorizes the following practitioners to prescribe controlled substances if they have a valid DEA registration number:

        a. Medical Doctors licensed under Chapter 458 (M.D.)
        b. Osteopathic physicians licensed under Chapter 459 (D.O.)
        c. Dentists licensed under Chapter 466 (D.D.S. or D.M.D.)
        d. Podiatrists licensed under Chapter 461 (D.P.M.)
        e. Veterinarians licensed under Chapter 474 (D.V.M.)
        f. Certified Optometrists licensed under Chapter 463 (O.D.)

Note: Optometrists have a limited formulary that includes only 2 controlled substances: tramadol and acetaminophen with codeine No. 3. For general rules on prescriptions from certified optometrists, see Chapter 3, Section II. A.4.

STUDY TIP: Other healthcare practitioners such as chiropractors and naturopaths may be licensed by the Florida Department of Health, but they do not have prescriptive authority.

g. Physician Assistants licensed under Chapter 458 or 459 (PA)
Note: For general rules on prescriptions from Physician Assistants, see Chapter 3, Section II. A.2.
Controlled substance specific rules are as follows:
   (1) Authority to prescribe controlled substances must be delegated by supervising physician.
   (2) Schedule II controlled substances are limited to a 7-day supply.
   (3) PAs may not prescribe controlled substances in a pain management clinic.
   (4) PAs may not prescribe psychiatric mental health controlled substances for children younger than 18.
   (5) Additional requirements and restrictions on treatment of pain that apply to all prescribers of controlled substances are also applicable. *See Section VII. E. below.*

h. Advanced Practice Registered Nurses licensed under Chapter 464 (APRN)
Note: For general rules on prescriptions from APRNs, see Chapter 3, Section II. A.3.
Controlled substance specific rules are as follows:
   (1) Authority to prescribe controlled substances must be delegated by supervising physician.
   (2) Schedule II controlled substances are limited to a 7-day supply. This limitation does not apply to controlled substances that are psychiatric medication prescribed by psychiatric nurses.
   (3) May not prescribe controlled substances in a pain management clinic.
   (4) Except for psychiatric nurses, may not prescribe psychiatric mental health controlled substances for children younger than 18.
   (5) Additional requirements and restrictions on treatment of pain that apply to all prescribers of controlled substances are also applicable. *See Section VII. E. below.*

i. Psychiatric Nurses
   (1) A psychiatric nurse is defined as an advanced practice registered nurse licensed under § 464.012 who has a master's or doctoral degree in psychiatric

nursing, holds a national advanced practice certification as a psychiatric mental health advanced practice nurse, and has 2 years of post-master's clinical experience under the supervision of a physician.

(2) Not subject to the 7-day limitation for Schedule II controlled substances if the Schedule II controlled substances are psychiatric medications.
Note: This makes sense to allow for prescribing of Schedule II drugs for ADHD, such as methylphenidate, for more than a 7-day supply.

(3) May prescribe psychiatric controlled substances to children younger than 18.

(4) Additional requirements that apply to APRNs and restrictions and requirements on the treatment of pain that apply to all prescribers of controlled substances are also applicable. *See Section VII. E. below.*

2. Out-of-State Prescribers
    a. The FLCSA definition of "practitioner" does not specifically include practitioners in other states.
    b. However, the definition of "prescription" in the Florida Pharmacy Act includes orders or those transmitted by practitioners in other jurisdictions, but only if the pharmacist called upon to dispense such an order determines that the order is valid and necessary for treatment of a chronic or recurrent condition.
    c. Based on this, it appears that prescriptions from out-of-state practitioners for controlled substances may be filled if the pharmacist validates the prescription and it is for a chronic or recurring condition.

3. Out-of-Country Practitioners
    a. Controlled substances prescriptions—A practitioner in another country cannot have a DEA registration, therefore any prescription for a controlled substance issued in another country is not permitted.
    b. Non-controlled substance prescriptions—It is less clear for non-controlled substances, but as noted above, the definition of a prescription in the Florida Pharmacy Act only recognizes prescriptions from "other jurisdictions" if the drug is for a chronic condition. If "other jurisdictions" is interpreted to include other countries, then perhaps those prescriptions would be valid. If "other

jurisdictions" means other U.S. states and territories only, then those prescriptions are not valid. Without a definitive statement in the laws and rules that permits prescriptions from out of the country, it is likely that such prescriptions are not valid.
4. Telehealth Providers
   a. Telehealth is recognized in Florida and is regulated with specific standards of practice and recordkeeping requirements.
   b. Prescriptions from telehealth providers are valid assuming they are based on a valid practitioner-patient relationship.
   c. Telehealth providers may not prescribe controlled substances under Florida law unless the controlled substance is prescribed for the following:
      (1) The treatment of a psychiatric disorder;
      (2) Inpatient treatment at a hospital;
      (3) The treatment of a patient receiving hospice services; or
      (4) The treatment of a resident of a nursing home facility.
5. Designated Agents
   a. Can communicate a prescription for a C-III–C-V controlled substance but cannot authorize or prescribe.
   b. An authorized agent of the prescriber (employee or non-employee) may not verbally communicate emergency C-II prescriptions to a pharmacist. This task cannot be delegated.
   c. DEA requires that for non-employees of the prescriber to qualify as an agent of the prescriber, there must be a formal written appointment of the agent by the prescriber. This is important for facilities such as nursing homes, where the nurses may not be employees of the physician but may wish to call in a prescription to a pharmacy on behalf of a physician.

C. Mandatory Electronic Prescriptions for Controlled Substances
   1. Florida passed legislation in 2019 requiring that healthcare practitioners issue all prescriptions (including controlled substance prescriptions) electronically. Technically, the law only applies to healthcare practitioners who maintain a system of electronic health records, but that is nearly every practitioner today.

2. This requirement becomes effective upon renewal of the healthcare practitioner's license or by July 1, 2021, whichever is earlier.
3. Electronic prescriptions are not required when:
   a. The practitioner and the dispenser are the same entity;
   b. The prescription cannot be transmitted electronically under the most recently implemented version of the National Council for Prescription Drug Programs SCRIPT Standard;
   c. The practitioner has been issued a waiver by the department, not to exceed 1 year, due to demonstrated economic hardship, technology limitations that are not reasonably within the control of the practitioner, or another exceptional circumstance demonstrated by the practitioners;
   d. The practitioner reasonably determines that it would be impractical for the patient in question to obtain a medicinal drug prescribed by electronic prescription in a timely manner and such delay would adversely impact the patient's medical condition;
   e. The practitioner is prescribing a drug under a research protocol;
   f. The prescription is for a drug for which the federal Food and Drug Administration requires the prescription to contain elements that may not be included in electronic prescribing;
   g. The prescription is issued to an individual receiving hospice care or who is a resident of a nursing home facility; or
   h. The practitioner determines that it is in the best interest of the patient, or the patient determines that it is in his or her own best interest, to compare prescription drug prices among area pharmacies. The practitioner must document such determination in the patient's medical record.

STUDY TIP: Because of the many exceptions to the mandatory electronic prescription requirements, you may still see questions about written and verbal prescriptions for controlled substances on the MPJE.

D. Written Controlled Substance Prescriptions
  1. Must be manually signed by the practitioner and dated on the date issued.
  2. Must be written on a counterfeit-proof prescription pad obtained from a vendor approved by the Florida Department of Health. *Note: This does not apply to prescriptions written by veterinarians.* Counterfeit-proof prescription pads must meet specific requirements, including:
     a. The background color must be blue or green and resist reproduction.
     b. The pad or blank must be printed on artificial water-marked paper.
     c. The pad or blank must resist erasures and alterations.
     d. The word "void" or "illegal" must appear on any photocopy or other reproduction of the pad or blank.
     e. The prescription must contain specific information, including a unique tracking identification number for each order on the front of the counterfeit-proof prescription pad or blank.

STUDY TIP: Although most prescriptions will have to be issued electronically by July 1, 2021, there are enough exceptions to the mandatory electronic prescription requirement that you must know the requirements for written prescriptions, including counterfeit-proof prescription pads.

  3. A prescription for a controlled substance may not be issued on the same prescription blank with a prescription for a non-controlled drug.
  4. Must contain:
     a. The full name and address of the patient.
     b. The drug name, strength, and dosage form.
     c. The quantity prescribed.
        Note: Florida law requires that the quantity prescribed must be written numerically and textually (as a word). Example: Vicodin #20 (twenty). This is not required for electronic prescriptions. If the quantity is not written as a word, the pharmacist should call to verify the quantity.
     d. Directions for use.
     e. Number of refills authorized, if any (not for Schedule II).
     f. The name, address, and DEA number of the practitioner.

      g. If written for a Schedule II prescription to be filled at a later date, the earliest date on which a pharmacy may fill a prescription.
      h. Florida law requires all written controlled substance prescriptions filled to have a prescription number, the initials of the pharmacist filling the prescription, and the date filled. *See FCSA § 893.04(c)5. and 6.*

E. Verbal, Fax, and Electronic Prescriptions
   1. Verbal prescriptions are not valid for Schedule II controlled substances unless it is an emergency.
   2. Verbal prescriptions are valid for Schedule III–V controlled substances.
   3. Florida does not allow a pharmacist to dispense more than a 30-day supply for a Schedule III controlled substance from a verbal prescription. *See FLCSA § 893.05(2)(e)*

STUDY TIP: This law was put into place when hydrocodone combination products were still Schedule III drugs. Since then, they have been rescheduled into Schedule II and therefore cannot be verbal except in an emergency, but the law is still in place. This is a law that is unique to Florida and could easily be the subject of an MPJE question.

BONUS STUDY TIP: If a verbal Schedule III prescription is limited to a 30-day supply, can a pharmacist dispense any authorized refills that go beyond the 30 days? The law is unclear on this, but the Florida Board of Pharmacy clarified this issue in a declaratory statement. The Board's opinion is that authorized refills may be dispensed but that each refill must not exceed a 30-day supply.

---

   4. Fax prescriptions are valid for Schedule III–V controlled substances but must have the prescriber's original signature. Electronic signatures are not valid on faxed controlled substance prescriptions. Faxes for Schedule II controlled substances are only allowed in limited circumstances. *See Section VII. B below.*
   5. Electronic prescriptions for controlled substances (including Schedule II) are valid if both the prescriber's computer and the pharmacy's computer meet all DEA security requirements.

STUDY TIP: Electronic prescriptions must be from the prescriber's computer to the pharmacy's computer. Faxes are not considered electronic prescriptions.

VII. Schedule II Prescriptions
  A. General
  1. Schedule II prescriptions must be either written or electronically submitted.
  2. Verbal prescriptions for Schedule II drugs are not permitted except in an emergency. *See C. Emergency Dispensing of a Verbal Schedule II Prescription below.*
  3. Schedule II prescriptions cannot be refilled.
  4. There is no time limit under federal law as to when a Schedule II prescription must be filled after being issued by the practitioner. However, under Florida law, all prescriptions (including Schedule II controlled substances) must be filled within one year after the date issued or the first date authorized to fill.

STUDY TIP: This creates the odd situation where Schedule II prescriptions are technically valid for up to one year, but Schedule III–V prescriptions are valid for only 6 months. Even though a Schedule II prescription may be technically valid for one year, pharmacists must use professional judgment and exercise their corresponding responsibility before dispensing a controlled substance prescription to ensure it is valid.

  5. Quantity Limits on Schedule II Prescriptions
      a. There is not a specific quantity limit for all Schedule II controlled substances on a single prescription under federal or Florida law.
      b. All prescribers in Florida are subject to quantity limits when prescribing Schedule II opioid products for acute pain. *See Section VII.E. below.*
      c. PAs and APRNs may only prescribe up to a 7-day supply of Schedule II controlled substance. There is an exception for psychiatric nurses.
      d. There is a 90-day supply limit when a practitioner issues multiple Schedule II prescriptions the same day. *See 6. below.*
      e. Although there is technically no quantity limit on a single controlled substance prescription, pharmacists should exercise their corresponding responsibility on every prescription to ensure it is legitimate. Insurance plans or pharmacy policies may limit the amount that

may be filled on a single prescription, but these are not legal requirements.
6. Changing Information or Information Omitted
   a. DEA provided guidance to the profession and state boards of pharmacies in 2011 regarding information a pharmacist may add or change on a written Schedule II prescription. DEA stated that whether a pharmacist may make changes to a Schedule II prescription—such as adding the practitioner's DEA number, or correcting the patient's name or address—varies case by case based on the facts present. Thus, "DEA expects that when information is missing from or needs to be changed on a Schedule II controlled substance prescription, pharmacists use their professional judgment and knowledge of state and federal laws and policies to decide whether it is appropriate to make changes to that prescription." DEA also said pharmacists should rely on state rules and guidance in making any such changes.
   b. I was unable to find any guidance from the Florida Board of Pharmacy on this issue, but generally, pharmacists can change items such as drug strength, dosage form, quantity, or directions for use, provided the pharmacist:
      (1) Contacts the prescribing practitioner and receives verbal permission for the change.
      (2) Documents on the prescription that the change was authorized, the name or initials of the individual granting the authorization, and the pharmacist's initials.
   c. The items that a pharmacist generally cannot change even after calling the prescriber on a written Schedule II prescription include:
      (1) Name of the patient.
      (2) Name of the drug.
      (3) Name of the prescribing physician.
7. Multiple Prescriptions for Schedule II Drugs. (DEA Rule 21 CFR 1306.12(b)(1))
   a. DEA permits an individual practitioner to issue multiple Schedule II prescriptions on the same day, authorizing the patient to receive a total of no more than a 90-day supply of a Schedule II controlled substance.

Instructions indicating the earliest fill date on which the prescriptions can be filled must be on each prescription.
  b. This 90-day limit only applies when the prescriber is issuing multiple prescriptions for a Schedule II controlled substance on the same day, with instructions that some of the prescriptions are not to be filled until a later date. *Note: Logically, if there is no quantity limit for a single Schedule II prescription, then there is no reason for this rule. Technically, that is correct, but in this case DEA realized that because many insurance plans don't cover more than a 30-day supply of controlled substances, patients would need to go to the prescriber every month to get a new written prescription for any Schedule II controlled substance since they could not be called in. This was before electronic prescriptions were more prevalent. Rather than having prescribers postdate a prescription, which DEA has never allowed and still does not allow, this rule was adopted. When it adopted this rule, DEA limited the total quantity to 90 days, but it has still not placed a days' supply limit on a single controlled substance prescription.*

STUDY TIP: The rules for issuing multiple Schedule II prescriptions seem to cause much confusion with pharmacy students and pharmacists. Be sure you understand this concept. These are not considered refills.

B. Facsimile Prescriptions for Schedule II Controlled Substances
  1. Facsimiles are generally not valid for Schedule II prescriptions.
  2. However, DEA recognizes three exceptions where a facsimile can serve as the original written prescription:
   a. A practitioner prescribing a Schedule II narcotic for a patient undergoing home infusion/IV pain therapy;
   b. A practitioner prescribing a Schedule II controlled substance for patients in Long Term Care Facilities (LTCFs); and
   c. A practitioner prescribing a Schedule II narcotic for a patient in hospice care.
C. Emergency Dispensing of a Schedule II Controlled Substance Pursuant to a Verbal Prescription
  1. In an emergency situation, a practitioner may provide a verbal Schedule II prescription to a pharmacy.

STUDY TIP: Communication must be from the prescriber and not a designated agent.

2. Emergency means that the immediate administration of the drug is necessary for the proper treatment of the ultimate user, that no alternative treatment is available, and that it is not possible for the prescribing practitioner to provide a written prescription.
3. The quantity prescribed and dispensed is limited to the amount needed to treat the patient during the emergency period. Florida law is stricter and specifies that the quantity for an emergency verbal Schedule II prescription is limited to a 72-hour supply. *See FLCSA § 893.04(1)(f)*
4. The prescription order must be immediately reduced to writing by the pharmacist and contain all information except the practitioner's signature.
5. If the prescriber is not known to the pharmacist, the pharmacist must make a reasonable effort to determine that the phone authorization came from a valid practitioner.
6. Within 7 days after authorizing an emergency telephone prescription, the prescribing practitioner must furnish the pharmacist a signed or a valid electronic prescription for the controlled substance prescribed (if mailed, it must be postmarked within 7 days). The prescription should be marked, "Authorization for Emergency Dispensing."
7. If the prescriber fails to deliver a written or electronic prescription, the pharmacist must notify the nearest DEA office.

STUDY TIP: Remember, the quantity of a Schedule II prescription that may be prescribed verbally in an emergency is limited to a 72-hour supply under Florida law. That is different from federal law.

D. Partial Dispensing of a Schedule II Controlled Substance Prescription
   1. 72-Hour Rule
      a. If a pharmacist is unable to fill the entire quantity on a Schedule II controlled substance prescription, a partial quantity may be provided so long as the remaining quantity is provided within 72 hours.
      b. If the remaining quantity cannot be provided, the pharmacist must notify the prescriber.

2. 30-Day Rule
   a. Under the Comprehensive Addiction and Recovery Act (CARA) of 2016, federal law was modified in 2016 to allow partial fills of Schedule II controlled substances for up to 30 days if requested by the patient of the prescriber.
   b. The total quantity dispensed may not exceed the original quantity prescribed.
   c. This applies to written and electronic prescriptions, but not to emergency verbal Schedule II controlled substance prescriptions.
   Note: DEA has yet to update their partial fill regulations or Pharmacist Manual to reflect this change.
3. 60-Day Rule
   a. For terminally ill and LTCF patients, both federal and Florida law allow partial fills of Schedule II prescriptions as many times as needed as long as the partial fillings are recorded on the prescription or maintained in the pharmacy's computer system.
   b. All partial fills for terminally ill and LTCF patients must be completed within 60 days.

STUDY TIP: Be sure to understand the difference between a partial fill and a refill. Partial fills are not considered a full refill. Remember, there are no refills on a Schedule II controlled substance prescription.

E. Florida Restrictions on the Treatment of Acute Pain (Florida Statute 456.44)
   1. General Information
      a. In response to the opioid epidemic, in 2018 the Florida Legislature made major changes to the Florida Controlled Substances Act that, among other things, placed prescribing limits on certain Schedule II prescriptions.
      b. The major provisions of the law are summarized below, but helpful information, including Frequently Asked Questions, can be found at the Take Control of Controlled Substances website of the Florida Department of Health at *http://www.flhealthsource.gov/FloridaTakeControl*.
   2. Definitions
      a. Acute Pain—The normal, predicted, physiological, and time-limited response to an adverse chemical,

thermal, or mechanical stimulus associated with surgery, trauma, or acute illness. The term does not include pain related to:
- **(1)** Cancer;
- **(2)** A terminal condition (defined as a progressive disease or medical or surgical condition that causes significant functional impairment, is not considered by a treating physician to be reversible without the administration of life-sustaining procedures, and will result in death within one year after diagnosis if the condition runs its normal course);
- **(3)** Palliative care to provide relief of symptoms related to an incurable, progressive illness or injury; or
- **(4)** A traumatic injury with an Injury Severity Score of 9 or greater.

Note: This is somewhat counterintuitive, as treatment of a traumatic injury seems like it should be acute pain. However, the definition of "acute pain" specifically excludes traumatic injuries with an Injury Severity Score of 9 or greater.

    b. Chronic nonmalignant pain—Pain unrelated to cancer that persists beyond the usual course of disease or the injury that is the cause of the pain, or more than 90 days after surgery.

    c. Emergency opioid antagonist—Naloxone hydrochloride or any similar-acting drug that blocks the effects of opioids; that is administered outside the body; and that is approved by the FDA for the treatment of opioid overdose.

    d. Registrant—A physician, physician assistant, or advanced practice registered nurse who prescribes any controlled substance in Schedules II, III, or IV for the treatment of chronic non-malignant pain.

3. Prescription Requirements
    a. For the treatment of acute pain, a prescription for an opioid drug listed in Schedule II may not exceed a 3-day supply, except that a prescriber can prescribe a 7-day supply if:
- **(1)** The prescriber, in his or her professional judgment, believes that more than a 3-day supply of such an opioid is medically necessary to treat the patient's pain;

(2) The prescriber indicates "Acute Pain Exception" on the prescription; and
(3) The prescriber adequately documents in the patient's medical records the acute medical condition and lack of alternative treatment options that justify deviation from the 3-day supply limit.

STUDY TIP: This 3-day/7-day limit only applies to Schedule II opioids for the treatment of acute pain. It does not apply to all Schedule II drugs, nor does it apply to opioids not being prescribed for acute pain.

    b. For the treatment of pain other than acute pain, a prescriber must write "Non-acute Pain" on a prescription for an opioid drug listed in Schedule II.

STUDY TIP: "Acute Pain Exception" is only required on the prescription to increase the quantity from a 3-day supply to a 7-day supply for acute pain. "Non-acute Pain" is required on the prescription when treating other than acute pain so that neither the 3-day nor 7-day limits would apply.

    c. For the treatment of pain related to a traumatic injury with an Injury Severity Score of 9 or greater, a prescriber who prescribes a Schedule II controlled substance must concurrently prescribe an emergency opioid antagonist.

4. Pharmacy Frequently Asked Questions on Treatment of Pain
    a. If a prescriber forgets to write "Acute Pain Exception" or "Non-acute Pain" on a prescription for a Schedule II opioid, may the pharmacist confirm with the prescriber and annotate the prescription?
Yes, the pharmacist should follow their standard policies and procedures by contacting the prescriber to verify written information on the prescription. Any change should be promptly reduced to writing.
    b. Do prescribers need to write the words "Non-acute Pain" on a prescription for an opioid drug listed in Schedule II if the quantity is greater than a 7-day supply?
Yes, assuming the prescription is written for pain, any prescriptions for an opioid in Schedule II that is greater than a 7-day supply would have to be marked "Non-acute Pain."

- c. When a prescription is provided electronically, if a note is included or transmitted to the pharmacist that indicates "Acute Pain Exception" or "Non-acute Pain," will that meet the requirements of the law?
Yes, if the "note" is transmitted with or is part of the electronic prescription, then the note would be acceptable.
F. Additional Florida Restrictions for Schedule II Controlled Substances
  1. Dispensing Schedule II or III Controlled Substances (§ 465.0181)
  Note: This applies to both Schedule II and III controlled substances but is placed here for ease of learning.
     a. Only community pharmacies (including limited community pharmacy permits) can dispense Schedule II or III controlled substance prescriptions.
     b. This was put in place in the midst of the opioid crisis to eliminate most physician dispensing of these products.
     c. There are some exceptions in the dispensing practitioner statute. See § 465.0276 in Chapter 5, Section II.B.
  2. Identification Requirements (§ 465.0155(2))
  Note: This applies to all controlled substance prescriptions, not just Schedule II.
     a. Before dispensing a controlled substance to a person not known to the pharmacist, the pharmacist must require the person purchasing, receiving, or otherwise acquiring the controlled substance to present valid photographic identification.
     b. If the person does not have proper identification, the pharmacist may verify the validity of the prescription and the identity of the patient with the prescriber or his or her agent.
     c. Verification of health plan eligibility through a real-time inquiry or adjudication system is considered to be proper identification.

STUDY TIP: Does Florida require a photo identification for controlled substance prescriptions? Yes, if the person is not known to the pharmacist. However, a major exception is if the prescription was adjudicated through a health plan. This implies that for cash-paying patients it is required if the person is not known to the pharmacist. Also, if the patient does not have proper identification, the pharmacist can verify their identity through the prescriber, although it is unclear how that would work.

    3. All applicants for a pharmacy permit in Florida must include written policies and procedures for preventing controlled substance dispensing based on fraudulent representations or invalid practitioner-patient relationships.

VIII. Schedule III–V Prescriptions
Note: Several of the requirements below will no longer be applicable once the Florida requirements for mandatory electronic prescriptions go into effect. Because there are so many exceptions to those requirements, however, pharmacists need to know the requirements for written, faxed, and verbal Schedule III–V prescriptions.
  A. General Rules
    1. May be filled from written, verbal, and facsimile prescriptions.

STUDY TIP: Florida law restricts verbal prescriptions for Schedule III controlled substances to no more than a 30-day supply.

    2. May be filled from electronic prescriptions as long as all DEA security requirements are met.
    3. May be refilled as indicated on the original prescription up to 5 times or 6 months.

STUDY TIP: There is no limit on the number of partial fills that can be provided, so long as the total amount dispensed does not exceed the total number of dosage units authorized and it is within the 6-month time period. Some pharmacy computer systems count each partial fill as a refill and invalidate the prescription after 5 partial fills, but this is not legally accurate. These prescriptions are still valid if the full quantities for all refills authorized have not been dispensed within 6 months.

  B. Transfers
    1. Refills of Schedule III–V controlled substances may be transferred to another pharmacy on a onetime basis.
    2. If pharmacies share an electronic, real-time, online database of prescriptions, they may transfer up to the maximum number of refills permitted by law and the prescriber's authorization.

3. Only refills may be transferred. DEA rules do not permit a pharmacy to transfer an original controlled substance prescription that has been received at a pharmacy, but not yet filled, to another pharmacy. An exception to this is permitted by DEA policy that allows an original electronic prescription for a controlled substance (EPCS), including a Schedule II prescription, to be transferred to another pharmacy if both pharmacies have the capability to forward and receive the EPCS using an electronic sharing program. *Note: Florida law also allows transfers of original prescriptions and not just refills. See Chapter 4, Section III.F. Although the procedure in 3. above is allowed by DEA Policy and Florida law, some pharmacies may choose not to do this and some pharmacy computer systems do not have this capability.*

C. OTC Sale of Schedule V Products (exempt narcotics)
  1. The FCSA (and Florida law) allow certain Schedule V products to be purchased from a pharmacy without a prescription.
  2. These are mainly cough suppressant products containing small amounts of codeine, such as Robitussin AC and products for diarrhea containing small amounts of opium.
  3. The total quantity that may be sold to any one purchaser within a 48-hour time period may not exceed:
     a. 120 mg of codeine;
     b. 60 mg of dihydrocodeine;
     c. 30 mg of ethyl morphine; and
     d. 240 mg of opium.

STUDY TIP: Florida law limits these quantities by mg of the drug, while federal law limits these quantities by volume as follows: Not more than 240 cc (8 oz.) of opium and not more than 120 cc (4 oz.) of any other controlled substance (codeine, etc.). It is recommended to know both of these limits.

  4. Other requirements:
     a. Dispensing may only be made by a pharmacist and not by a non-pharmacist, even if under the supervision of a pharmacist (although after the pharmacist has made the dispensing and met recordkeeping requirements, the actual sale and delivery may be completed by a non-pharmacist).
     b. The purchaser must be at least 18 years of age and the pharmacist must require every purchaser not known

to the pharmacist to provide identification and proof of age.
   c. A bound record book must be maintained by the pharmacist that contains the name and address of the purchaser, the name and quantity of the controlled substance purchased, the date of the purchase, and the name or initials of the pharmacist who dispensed the product to the purchaser.

STUDY TIP: Although this is technically allowed, most pharmacies do not sell these products without a prescription, but the law is still on the books and it is still listed in the MPJE competency statements.

D. Additional Florida Requirements for Schedule III–V Controlled Substances
   1. Identification Requirements (§ 465.0155(2)):
      Note: This applies to all controlled substance prescriptions, not just Schedule III–V.
      a. Before dispensing a controlled substance to a person not known to the pharmacist, the pharmacist must require the person purchasing, receiving, or otherwise acquiring the controlled substance to present valid photographic identification.
      b. If the person does not have proper identification, the pharmacist may verify the validity of the prescription and the identity of the patient with the prescriber or his or her agent.
      c. Verification of health plan eligibility through a real-time inquiry or adjudication system is considered to be proper identification.
   2. All applicants for a pharmacy permit in Florida must include written policies and procedures for preventing controlled substance dispensing based on fraudulent representations or invalid practitioner-patient relationships.

IX. **Methadone, Opiate Dependence, Naloxone, and Methamphetamine Controls**
   A. Prescribing and Dispensing of Certain Narcotic Drugs
      1. Methadone is used both for the treatment of severe pain and in the detoxification and maintenance of narcotic addicts in registered narcotic treatment programs.

2. While any pharmacy can stock methadone, it can only legally be dispensed as an analgesic (for pain treatment).
3. DEA has requested manufacturers and wholesalers to voluntarily restrict sales of methadone 40 mg to hospitals and narcotic treatment clinics only; no sales to retail pharmacies are allowed.
4. Methadone (or any other drug) cannot be dispensed for the maintenance or detoxification of addicts unless it is provided through a registered narcotic treatment center.
5. Narcotic treatment facilities may administer and dispense (but not prescribe) narcotic drugs to a narcotic-dependent person for detoxification or maintenance treatment.
    a. Short-term detoxification means dispensing of a narcotic drug in decreasing doses for a period not to exceed 30 days.
    b. Long-term detoxification means dispensing of a narcotic drug to a narcotic-dependent person in decreasing doses in excess of 30 days but not in excess of 180 days.

STUDY TIP: Make sure you understand that a narcotic treatment program is a specific type of DEA registration that permits the administration and dispensing of methadone, but those practitioners may not write prescriptions such as methadone for treating addiction that can be filled at a pharmacy. Pharmacies may only dispense prescriptions for methadone for pain. It is acceptable to dispense a prescription for methadone as part of a formal pain management program in which a patient is switched to methadone to control or gradually reduce dosage of other narcotics, but methadone cannot be dispensed from a pharmacy solely as a treatment for opioid dependency.

6. A physician who is not part of a narcotic treatment program may administer (not prescribe) narcotic drugs (e.g., methadone) to an addicted individual for not more than a 3-day period until the individual can be enrolled in a narcotic treatment program.
7. A hospital that is not part of a narcotic treatment program may administer narcotics to a drug-dependent person for either detoxification or maintenance therapy if the patient is being treated in the hospital for a condition other than the addiction.

B. Medication Assisted Treatment (MAT) for Opiate Dependence
    1. The Drug Addiction Treatment Act of 2000 (DATA 2000) allows office-based, specially trained practitioners to

prescribe certain narcotic Schedule III–V drugs to treat opiate dependence through a risk management program outside of a narcotic treatment facility.
2. A practitioner authorized to prescribe under the Act, called a DATA-waived practitioner, can apply for a DATA 2000 waiver if they meet specific criteria. The waiver is provided by the Substance Abuse and Mental Health Services Administration (SAMHSA), and the practitioner is provided an identification or "X" code that must be included with the prescriber's DEA number. Pharmacists can verify a practitioner's DATA waiver at the SAMHSA website's Buprenorphine Pharmacy Lookup.
3. The only drugs that may be dispensed under this program are Subutex® (buprenorphine) and Suboxone® (buprenorphine/naloxone combination). These drugs, both Schedule III controlled substances, are available in sublingual form and may be dispensed by a pharmacy upon a prescription from a qualified practitioner.
4. A DATA-waived physician may be allowed to treat up to 30, 100, or 275 patients, depending on his or her authorization. A DATA-waived APRN or PA may initially treat up to 30 patients. After one year, a DATA-waived APRN or PA may apply for authorization to treat up to 100 patients.

STUDY TIP: A DATA-waived practitioner can treat opioid addiction and prescribe MAT drugs (buprenorphine and buprenorphine/naloxone) from his or her office. They do not need to work at or be registered as a Narcotic Treatment Program. Likewise, a practitioner that is part of a Narcotic Treatment Program cannot automatically prescribe MAT drugs to be filled at a pharmacy. They would also need to be a DATA-waived practitioner.

C. Dispensing of Naloxone in Florida (Florida Statue 381.887)
Note: Although naloxone is not a controlled substance, it is included in this chapter since it concerns treatment of opioid addiction.
1. This section of the Public Health Act permits a Florida-licensed pharmacist to dispense an emergency opioid antagonist such as naloxone based on a non-patient specific standing order for an auto-injection delivery system or intranasal application delivery system.

2. The State Surgeon General issued a statewide naloxone standing order for all pharmacies in Florida that authorizes the dispensing of naloxone to emergency responders.
3. Pharmacies would need to have a separate standing order from a physician in order to dispense naloxone to patients, caregivers, or others.
4. A pharmacist, acting in good faith and exercising reasonable care, is not subject to discipline or other adverse action under any professional licensure statute or rule and is immune from any civil or criminal liability as a result of dispensing an emergency opioid antagonist.

D. The Combat Methamphetamine Epidemic Act of 2005
1. This law was passed by Congress to further control the sale of OTC products containing precursor chemicals used in the illicit manufacturing of methamphetamine.
2. The law classifies all products (including multiple-ingredient products) containing ephedrine, pseudoephedrine, and phenylpropanolamine as "listed chemical products." *Note: Since this law was passed, ephedrine and phenylpropanolamine products have all been removed from the market by FDA, so the law really only impacts pseudoephedrine products.*
3. Products containing a "listed chemical" are subject to the following requirements:
    a. Display Restrictions—Although the products may be sold by any retailer, covered products must be placed behind a counter (not necessarily a pharmacy counter) or, if located on the selling floor, in a locked cabinet.
    b. Retail Sales Limits—Sales of covered products to an individual are limited to 3.6 g of the base product per day and 9 g of the base product per 30 days. Many states have sales limits per transaction.
    c. For pseudoephedrine HCL, the daily limit of 3.6 g of base product equals:
        (1) 146 of the 30 mg tablets
        (2) 73 of the 60 mg tablets
        (3) 36 of the 120 mg tablets
    d. Product Packaging—Covered products (other than liquids including gel caps) must either be in blister or unit-dose packaging.

4. Recordkeeping Requirements:
   a. Retailer must maintain an electronic or written logbook that identifies the products by name, quantity sold, names and addresses of purchasers, and dates and times of sales.
   b. There is an exception for the logbook requirement for individual sales of a single "convenience" package of less than 60 mg of pseudoephedrine.
   c. Purchaser must present a photo identification issued by a state or federal government, must sign logbook, and must enter his or her name, address, and date and time of sale.
   d. Retailer must verify that the name entered in the logbook corresponds to the customer identification.
5. Florida Requirements:
   a. Florida law requires the purchaser to be at least 18 years old.
   b. Florida law requires pharmacies to use the approved Florida Department of Law Enforcement electronic recordkeeping system to meet the recordkeeping requirements. The electronic system provides real-time tracking of nonprescription sales of these products. A pharmacy can request an exemption from the electronic recordkeeping system if it maintains a sales volume of less than 72 g of base product in a 30-day period. *See FLCSA § 893.1495(5)(b)*
6. Employee Training:
   a. Employers certify that employees who deal directly with customers have undergone training to ensure they understand the requirements of the law.
   b. DEA requirements for self-certification and training can be found at *www.deadiversion.usdoj.gov/meth/index.html*.
7. Mail Service Limitations:
   a. Mail service companies must confirm the identity of purchasers.
   b. Sales are limited to 7.5 g per 30-day period.
8. Mobile Retail Vendors ("flea markets"):
   a. Product must be placed in a locked cabinet.
   b. Sales are limited to no more than 7.5 g of base product per customer per 30 days.

X. E-FORCSE™: The Florida Prescription Drug Monitoring Program (PDMP)
   A. General Information
      1. The Electronic Online Reporting of Controlled Substances Evaluation program or E-FORCSE™ is Florida's Prescription Drug Monitoring Program (PDMP). It is run by the Florida Department of Health. Rules from the Department of Health for the PDMP can be found under Florida Administrative Code, Chapter 64K-1.
      2. The purpose of the PDMP is to provide the information that will be collected in the database to healthcare practitioners to guide their decisions in prescribing and dispensing these highly abused prescription drugs.
      3. Information in the PDMP database is not discoverable or admissible in any civil or administrative action, except in an investigation and disciplinary proceeding by the Department of Health or the appropriate regulatory board. *See FLCSA § 893.055(7)(c)*
      4. The Florida PDMP is part of NABP's PMP InterConnect, allowing pharmacists to perform queries of a patient's controlled substance use in most other states.
   B. Mandatory Use
      1. Pharmacists, prescribers, and dispensers, or their designees, are required to access and consult the PDMP to review a patient's controlled substance dispensing history each time a controlled substance is prescribed or dispensed. *See FLCSA § 893.055(8) FAC Rule 64K-1.003(1)(f)(2)*

STUDY TIP: For pharmacists, the PDMP must be consulted for both new prescriptions and refills for controlled substances.

---

      2. Accessing and consulting the PDMP is not required:
         a. For patients under 16 years of age; and
         b. When prescribing or dispensing of a controlled substance to a patient who has been admitted to hospice.
         c. For non-narcotics in Schedule V. This would include:
            (1) pregabalin (Lyrica®);
            (2) brivaracetam (Brivact®);
            (3) lacosamide (Vimpat®); and
            (4) ezogabine (Potiga®)—this product is no longer on the market.

3. Accessing and consulting the PDMP is also not required:
   a. When the system is nonoperational as determined by the FDOH; or
   b. When the system cannot be accessed because of a temporary technological or electrical failure.
4. A prescriber or dispenser, or their designee, who does not consult the PDMP for any of the reasons in 3. above shall document the reason and shall not prescribe or dispense greater than a 3-day supply of a controlled substance to the patient.

C. Reporting Requirements
   1. Each time a controlled substance is dispensed to an individual in the state, the controlled substance must be reported through the PDMP system as soon thereafter as possible, but no later than the close of the next business day after the day the controlled substance is dispensed, unless an extension is approved by the department for cause as determined by rule. See FLCSA § 893.055(3)
   2. Extensions of time to report the dispensing of a controlled substance may be granted for no more than 30 days, upon request to the program by any dispenser unable to submit data by electronic means, if the dispenser provides evidence of having suffered a mechanical or electronic failure or cannot report for reasons beyond the control of the dispenser or if the system is unable to receive submissions.
   3. Exemptions from Reporting
      a. All acts of administration.
      b. The dispensing of a controlled substance in the healthcare system of the Department of Corrections.
      c. The dispensing of a controlled substance to a person under the age of 16.
      d. Pharmacies and registered dispensing practitioners that do not dispense controlled substances in or into this state must submit a "Notification of Exemption From Reporting," and must renew the exemption every two years when renewing their pharmacy permit.
   4. A dispenser that has no dispensing transactions to report for the preceding business day must submit a zero activity report as described in the "Data Submission Dispenser Guide."

5. Dispensing information with errors or omissions shall be corrected and resubmitted by the reporting dispenser within one business day of receiving electronic or written notice from the program manager or support staff of the error or omission.
6. The following information must be reported by a pharmacy:
   a. Name of the prescribing practitioner
   b. Practitioner's DEA number
   c. Practitioner's National Provider Identification (NPI) number
   d. Date prescription was issued
   e. Date prescription was filled
   f. Method of payment (cash, insurance, etc.)
   g. Name, address, telephone number, and date of birth of person for whom the prescription was written
   h. Name, NDC number, quantity, and strength of the controlled substance dispensed
   i. Name, DEA number, pharmacy permit number, and address of the pharmacy
   j. Whether prescription was an initial or refill and the number of refills ordered
   k. Name of the individual picking up the controlled substance prescription and type of identification provided

STUDY TIP: This information is reported electronically, but you should know what is required to be reported and when it is required to be reported for purposes of the MPJE.

D. Access and Privacy of PDMP Data
   1. Pharmacists, prescribers, and dispensers licensed in Florida may directly access the information in the PDMP by registering at *https://florida.pmpaware.net/login*.
   2. Pharmacists, prescribers, and dispensers may appoint a designee to access the PDMP to request and receive information.
      a. A designee must review the "PMP AWARxE Requestor User Support Manual" and the "Information Security and Privacy Training Course for Designees" prior to registering and complete the "Designee Certification Form." The designee must provide a printed copy of the

"Designee Certification Form" to the designating prescriber or dispenser.
   b. A designee will not have access to the PDMP until the designating prescriber or dispenser affirmatively accepts responsibility for the designee and links the designee to a pharmacy, prescriber, or dispenser account.
   c. Registered designees who do not access E-FORCSE® for a period in excess of six months will be deactivated. Deactivated designees may reapply for access.
3. PDMP data is confidential and considered protected health information.
4. A prescriber or dispenser, or his or her designee, may access the PDMP only for the purpose of reviewing the information related to a patient of the prescriber or dispenser.
5. Law enforcement agencies do not have direct access to the PDMP, but they may request information from the PDMP for an active investigation from the Department of Health if they have entered into a user agreement with the department.

STUDY TIP: A pharmacy cannot provide information from the PDMP to a law enforcement officer. A law enforcement agency would have to request information directly from the PDMP program at the Department of Health and only for an active investigation. Although it is similar information, a law enforcement officer can request a pharmacy to produce a summary record of controlled substances dispensed in the last 60 days from a specific prescriber or to a specific patient from a pharmacy pursuant to Rule 64B16-27.831(8).

CHAPTER THREE
Florida Laws—Part 1
Overview, Prescriptive Authority, Board of Pharmacy, Definitions, and Licensure

CHAPTER THREE
Florida Laws—Part 1
Overview, Prescriptive Authority, Board of Pharmacy, Definitions, and Licensure

I. Florida Laws Impacting Pharmacy Practice

This book does not cover every law and rule governing the practice of pharmacy in Florida, but instead highlights those most applicable to the MPJE Competency Statements. Rather than reviewing the laws and rules in order, this book, where possible, groups statutes and rules by topic. For most topics, a reference is provided to the specific statute or rule. This book summarizes and explains those provisions but may not always include the entire statutory or rule language. Often, the statutory or rule language is annotated to make it easier to understand, and the "notes" provide further explanation. The reader is advised to read all the laws and rules that apply in Florida.

The following are the most important provisions of Florida laws and rules relating to the practice of pharmacy.

A. Statutes (Laws)
 1. Chapter 456 Health Professions and Occupations
 Note: This is the general chapter for all health professions, but not all provisions of this chapter apply to pharmacists. Only those provisions in this chapter that specifically indicate they are applicable to persons licensed under Chapter 465 would apply to pharmacists. For example, Section 456.031 requires continuing education on domestic violence for several healthcare professionals, but that requirement does not apply to pharmacists.
 2. Chapter 465 Florida Pharmacy Act (FPA)
 3. Chapter 893 Florida Controlled Substances Act (FLCSA)
 4. Chapter 499 Florida Food, Drug and Cosmetics Act (FLFDCA)
 Note: Chapter 499 is administered by the Florida Department of Business and Professional Regulation (DBPR) and primarily applies to manufacturers and wholesale distributors, although some provisions may impact a pharmacy.

B. Rules—Florida Administrative Code
 1. Chapter 64B16-26 Pharmacists Licensure
 2. Chapter 64B16-27 Pharmacy Practice

3. Chapter 64B16-28 Permits
4. Chapter 64B16-29 Animal Control Shelter Permits
5. Chapter 64B16-30 Disciplinary Guidelines
6. Chapter 64B16-31 Collaborative Practice and Test and Treat Certifications
7. Chapter 64B16-32 Nonresident Pharmacies

C. Additional Helpful Information
1. The Florida Board of Pharmacy website (floridaspharmacy.gov) contains useful information for both practicing pharmacists and those seeking licensure in Florida. The website includes links to all statutes and rules as well as helpful information in the "Resources" section of the website.
2. The most current information from the Florida Board of Pharmacy can be obtained from the "Latest News" section of the website or by subscribing to updates via email.
3. Information on Board meetings is also provided, including agendas and minutes to stay informed on new rules being proposed and discussed.
4. Some additional study resources are the inspection forms for pharmacies, which can be found at the Florida Department of Health website. These forms cite specific portions of the laws and rules the inspectors look for when inspecting pharmacies, which can also be helpful when studying for the MPJE.

II. Prescriptive Authority and Scope of Practice

A. Prescriptive Authority
1. Practitioners with Independent Authority
   a. Allopathic physicians (M.D.) licensed under Chapter 458
   b. Osteopathic physicians (D.O.) licensed under Chapter 459
   c. Dentists licensed under Chapter 466
   d. Podiatrists licensed under Chapter 461
   e. Certified optometrists licensed under Chapter 463
   f. Veterinarians licensed under Chapter 474
2. Physician Assistants—Dependent Prescriptive Authority
   a. A supervising physician may delegate to a prescribing Physician Assistant only such authorized medicinal drugs as are used in the supervising physician's practice.
   b. Physician Assistants may not prescribe:
      (1) Psychiatric mental health controlled substances for children younger than 18 years of age;

        (2) General, spinal, or epidural anesthetics; or
        (3) Radiographic contrast materials.
    c. Controlled substance restrictions:
        (1) Schedule II controlled substances are limited to a 7-day supply.
        (2) Controlled substances may not be prescribed in a pain management clinic.
        (3) Other restrictions on prescribing Schedule II opioids for pain are also applicable. *See details in Chapter 2*
    d. In a hospital practice, a Physician Assistant may write orders for any medication.
3. Advanced Practice Registered Nurses (APRNs)—Dependent Prescriptive Authority
    a. May prescribe any drug based on a written protocol from a supervising physician.
    b. Controlled substance restrictions:
        (1) Schedule II controlled substances are limited to a 7-day supply. This limitation does not apply to controlled substances that are psychiatric medication prescribed by psychiatric nurses.
        (2) May not prescribe controlled substances in a pain management clinic.
        (3) Except for psychiatric nurses, may not prescribe psychiatric mental health controlled substances for children younger than 18.
        (4) Other restrictions on prescribing Schedule II opioids for pain are also applicable. *See details in Chapter 2*
    c. Psychiatric nurses:
        (1) A psychiatric nurse is defined as an advanced practice registered nurse licensed under § 464.012 who has a master's or doctoral degree in psychiatric nursing, holds a national advanced practice certification as a psychiatric mental health advanced practice nurse, and has 2 years of post-master's clinical experience under the supervision of a physician.
        (2) Not subject to the 7-day limitation for Schedule II controlled substances if the Schedule II controlled substances are psychiatric medications.
        (3) May prescribe psychiatric controlled substances to children younger than 18.

4. Certified Optometrists—Independent Authority but Limited Formulary
   a. Certified optometrists may administer and prescribe ocular pharmaceutical agents from an approved formulary for the diagnosis and treatment of ocular conditions of the human eye and its appendages without the use of surgery or other invasive techniques.

FORMULARY OF TOPICAL OCULAR PHARMACEUTICAL AGENTS THAT MAY BE PRESCRIBED BY CERTIFIED OPTOMETRISTS

(1) CYCLOPLEGIC AND MYDRIATICS
   (a) Atropine sulfate—1% (solution and ointment);
   (b) Phenylepherine HCl—2.5%;
   (c) Cyclopentolate HCl—0.5%, 1%;
   (d) Scopolamine HBr—0.25%;
   (e) Homatropine HBr—2%, 5%;
   (f) Tropicamide—0.5%, 1%; and
   (g) Hydroxyamphetamine HBr—1% plus tropicamide—0.25%.

(2) LOCAL ANESTHETICS
   (a) Tetracaine—0.5%;
   (b) Proparacaine HCl—0.5%; and
   (c) Benoxinate HCl—0.4% (in combination with fluorescein).

(3) DIAGNOSTIC PRODUCTS
   Fluorescein paper strips—1 mg, 9 mg per strip.

(4) ANTIBACTERIAL
   (a) Erythromycin—0.5%;
   (b) Bacitracin—400 units/g, 500 units/g (ointment alone and in combination);
   (c) Polymyxin—10,000 units/g (only in combination);
   (d) Neomycin—1.75 mg/g, 1.75 mg/ml, 3.50 mg/g (only in combination);
   (e) Gentamicin—0.3% (solution and ointment);
   (f) Tobramycin—0.3% (solution and ointment in combination);
   (g) Gramicidin—0.025 mg/ml (only in combination);
   (h) Ciprofloxacin HCl—0.3% (solution and ointment);
   (i) Trimethoprim—1 mg/ml (only in combination);
   (j) Ofloxaxin—0.3%;

- (k) Levofloxacin—1.5%;
- (l) Gatifloxacin—0.5%;
- (m) Moxifloxacin—0.5%;
- (n) Sodium sulfacetamide—10% (alone and in combination);
- (o) Azithromycin—1%; and
- (p) Besifloxacin Ophthalmic Suspension—0.6%.

(5) **NONSTEROIDAL AND STEROIDAL ANTI-INFLAMMATORY AGENTS**
- (a) Medrysone—1%;
- (b) Prednisolone acetate—0.12%, 0.125%, 0.2%, 0.5%, 0.6%, 1% (alone and in combination);
- (c) Prednisolone sodium phosphate—0.125%, 0.25%, 1% (alone and in combination);
- (d) Flurometholone—0.1%, 0.25% (suspension and ointment, alone and in combination);
- (e) Dexamethasone—0.1%, 1% (alone and in combination);
- (f) Dexamethasone sodium phosphate—0.1% (solution and ointment);
- (g) Fluorometholone acetate—0.1%;
- (h) Rimexolone—1%;
- (i) Loteprednol etabonate—0.2%, 0.5% (alone and in combination);
- (j) Diclofenac sodium—0.1%;
- (k) Ketorolac tromethamine—0.5%;
- (l) Hydrocortisone—1% (only in combination);
- (m) Bromfenac—0.09%;
- (n) Nepafenac—0.1%;
- (o) Difluprednate opthalmic emulsion—0.05%; and
- (p) Loteprednol etabonate ophthalmic suspension—1%.

(6) **ANTIHISTAMINES, MAST CELL STABILIZERS, AND ANTI-ALLERGY AGENTS**
- (a) Cromolyn sodium—4%;
- (b) Lodoxamide tromethamine—0.1%;
- (c) Olopatadine HCl—0.7%;
- (d) Nedocromil sodium—2%;
- (e) Azelastine HCl—0.05%;
- (f) Pemirolast potassium—0.1%;
- (g) Epinastine HCl—0.05%;
- (h) Bepotastine besilate—1.5%; and
- (i) Alcaftadine—0.25%.

(7) ANTIVIRAL AGENTS
    (a) Trifluridine—1%;
    (b) Ganciclovir—0.15%; and
    (c) Povidone-iodine ophthalmic solution—5%.

(8) ANTI-GLAUCOMA AGENTS
    (a) Beta Blockers
        1. Betaxolol HCl—0.25%, 0.5%;
        2. Levobunolol HCl—0.25%, 0.5%;
        3. Metipranolol HCl—0.3%;
        4. Timolol maleate or hemihydrate—0.25%, 0.5% (solution and gel, alone and in combination); and
        5. Carteolol HCl—1%.
    (b) Miotics, Direct-acting
        1. Carbachol—0.75%, 1.5%, 3%;
        2. Pilocarpine HCl—0.5%, 1%, 2%, 4%; and
        3. Pilocarpine gel—4%.
    (c) Prostaglandins
        1. Latanoprost—0.005%;
        2. Bimatoprost—0.03%;
        3. Travoprost—0.004%;
        4. Tafluprost—0.0015%;
        5. Unoprostone Isoprophyl—0.15%; and
        6. Latanoprostene Bunod Ophthalmic Solution—0.024%.
    (d) Alpha2 Adrenergic Agonist
        1. Brimonidine tartrate—0.15%, 0.2%; and
        2. Apraclonidine HCl—0.5%.
    (e) Carbonic Anhydrase Inhibitors (CAIs)
        1. Brinzolamide—1%; and
        2. Dorzolamide HCl—2% (alone and in combination).
    (f) Rho Kinase Inhibitor—Netarsudil—0.02%.

(9) MISCELLANEOUS
    (a) Hydroxypropyl cellulose ophthalmic insert;
    (b) Dapiprazole—0.5%;
    (c) Cyclosporine emulsion—0.05%;
    (d) Polyvinyl pyrrolidone—drops 2%;
    (e) Bimatoprost—0.03%;
    (f) Natamycin Opthalmic Suspension—5%;
    (g) Lifitegrast ophthalmic solution—5%; and
    (h) Cyclosporine 0.09% Opthalmic Solution.

b. Certified optometrists can also prescribe certain oral drugs after completing additional training.

FORMULARY OF ORAL DRUGS THAT MAY BE PRESCRIBED BY CERTIFIED OPTOMETRISTS

(1) **The following analgesics or their generic or therapeutic equivalents, which may not be administered or prescribed for more than 72 hours without consultation with a physician licensed under Chapter 458 or Chapter 459 and who is skilled in diseases of the eye:**
   (i) Tramadol hydrochloride.
   (ii) Acetaminophen 300 mg with No. 3 codeine phosphate 30 mg.

(2) **The following antibiotics or their generic or therapeutic equivalents:**
   (i) Amoxicillin with or without clavulanic acid.
   (ii) Azithromycin.
   (iii) Erythromycin.
   (iv) Dicloxacillin.
   (v) Doxycycline/Tetracycline.
   (vi) Keflex.
   (vii) Minocycline.

(3) **The following antivirals or their generic or therapeutic equivalents:**
   (i) Acyclovir.
   (ii) Famciclovir.
   (iii) Valacyclovir.

(4) **The following oral anti-glaucoma agents or their generic or therapeutic equivalents, which may not be administered or prescribed for more than 72 hours:**
   (i) Acetazolamide.
   (ii) Methazolamide.

B. Telehealth
   1. Telehealth is recognized in Florida and is regulated with specific standards of practice and recordkeeping requirements.
   2. Out-of-state healthcare practitioners must be registered with the Florida Department of Health to perform telehealth services for patients in Florida.

3. Prescriptions from telehealth providers are valid, assuming they are based on a valid practitioner-patient relationship. However, telehealth providers may not prescribe controlled substances unless the controlled substance is prescribed for the following:
   a. The treatment of a psychiatric disorder;
   b. Inpatient treatment at a hospital;
   c. The treatment of a patient receiving hospice services; or
   d. The treatment of a resident of a nursing home facility.

C. Standards for Prescribing of Obesity Drugs
   1. The Florida Board of Medicine has a rule that requires very specific procedures for the prescribing of obesity drugs (Rule 64B8-9.012).
   2. The rule requires that prescriptions or orders for any drug, synthetic compound, nutritional supplement, or herbal treatment for the purpose of assisting in weight loss be in writing and signed by the prescribing physician. It states that initial prescriptions or orders of this type shall not be called into a pharmacy by the physician or by an agent of the physician.
   3. This rule has been in place since 1998, before electronic prescriptions even existed. There has always been confusion about the rule since it says only the "initial" prescription had to be in writing, which implies that subsequent prescriptions or refills could be provided over the phone, but, to my knowledge, this has never been clarified. The other issue is, since it was written prior to the use electronic prescriptions, it only prohibits the "calling in" of initial prescriptions. The rule is clearly outdated, particularly since Florida has mandated electronic prescriptions; but as of the date of publication of this book, the rule has not been repealed or modified, so it is included here.

D. Mandatory Electronic Prescriptions
   1. As discussed in Chapter 2, Florida now requires all prescriptions be transmitted electronically unless certain exceptions are met.
   2. Those exceptions include:
      a. The practitioner and the dispenser are the same entity;
      b. The prescription cannot be transmitted electronically under the most recently implemented version of the National Council for Prescription Drug Programs SCRIPT Standard;

      c. The practitioner has been issued a waiver by the department, not to exceed 1 year, due to demonstrated economic hardship, technology limitations that are not reasonably within the control of the practitioner, or another exceptional circumstance demonstrated by the practitioner;
      d. The practitioner reasonably determines that it would be impractical for the patient in question to obtain a medicinal drug prescribed by electronic prescription in a timely manner and such delay would adversely impact the patient's medical condition;
      e. The practitioner is prescribing a drug under a research protocol;
      f. The prescription is for a drug for which the federal Food and Drug Administration requires the prescription to contain elements that may not be included in electronic prescribing;
      g. The prescription is issued to an individual receiving hospice care or who is a resident of a nursing home facility; or
      h. The practitioner determines that it is in the best interest of the patient, or the patient determines that it is in his or her own best interest, to compare prescription drug prices among area pharmacies. The practitioner must document such determination in the patient's medical record.

E. Pharmacists' Orders for Certain Medicinal Drugs
  1. Pharmacists are not recognized as healthcare practitioners with prescriptive authority, but they do have limited authority to independently order and dispense certain medicinal drugs to patients.
  2. These drugs must be dispensed by the pharmacist who ordered the drug. Pharmacists cannot issue a prescription to be filled by another pharmacist or at another pharmacy.
  3. See § 465.186 in Chapter 4, Section A. for details.

F. Miscellaneous Prescriptive Authority Issues
  1. Scope of Practice
      a. A physician (D.O. or M.D.) may legally prescribe a drug to treat any disease or illness. Although a pharmacist should exercise caution, it is legal to fill a prescription written outside of a physician's specialty, such as a

hypertension medication written by an orthopedic surgeon or an oncologist.
  b. Dentists, podiatrists, and veterinarians may only prescribe drugs used within their scope of practice. For example, a veterinarian cannot prescribe drugs for humans, and a prescription from a dentist for birth control pills would not be a valid prescription.
  c. Prescriptive authority for certified optometrists is restricted to the approved formulary.
2. Self-prescribing and Prescribing for Family Members
  a. The Florida Board of Medicine has indicated that self-prescribing of controlled substances is prohibited, but there is no specific law or rule that strictly forbids self-prescribing or prescribing for family members for non-controlled substances. In order to be a legal prescription, however, there must be a valid practitioner-patient relationship and the prescription must be issued in the usual course of professional practice.
  b. Self-prescribing or prescribing for an individual who is not a patient, as defined by having a valid patient chart or record, is not considered part of a practitioner's professional practice.
  c. Prescribing drugs outside of the course of professional practice is considered grounds for discipline of a physician in Florida.
  d. Pharmacists can also be disciplined for dispensing drugs when the pharmacist knows or has reason to believe a purported prescription is not based on a valid practitioner-patient relationship.

STUDY TIP: Even without a specific law that prohibits self-prescribing or prescribing for family members, pharmacists should exercise caution and only fill such prescriptions if they can validate that there is a valid practitioner-patient relationship and that the prescription was issued in the usual course of practice.

3. Retired or Deceased Practitioners
  a. One of the MPJE Competency Statements includes how to handle prescriptions after a practitioner retires or dies.
  b. Some states include specific rules or policies on how pharmacists should handle these situations, but Florida does not appear to address this topic.

      c. In the absence of specific guidance, this may be an opportunity to use the emergency refill rules. *See Chapter 4, Section III.H.*

> **STUDY TIP:** It is difficult to provide advice on how to answer a question on this topic in the absence of specific guidance from the state. The competency may be referring to DEA rule 1301.52(a), which states that a DEA registration terminates when a practitioner dies. From a strict legal view, it makes sense that any refills remaining on a prescription are no longer valid once a practitioner is deceased or retired. This may be the best legal answer, but it does not really take care of the patient. This topic has been in the MPJE Competencies long before states had emergency refill rules, which now provide a possible alternative, because a pharmacist certainly is unable to obtain refill authorization in this situation.

   4. Approved Drugs for Unapproved Uses—Off Label Use
      a. There is no law that prohibits a practitioner from prescribing, or a pharmacist from dispensing, an approved drug for a use that is not approved in the drug's labeling.
      b. Pharmacists should use their professional judgment in these situations and consider liability implications.
   5. Office Use Prescriptions
      a. Except for specific situations (such as dispensing naloxone based on a non-patient-specific standing order or a compounded prescription for office use), medicinal drugs can only be dispensed based on a patient-specific prescription.
      b. A prescription written "For Office Use" cannot be filled. A pharmacist can sell an original manufacturer's bottle of a prescription drug to a practitioner for use in his or her office, but cannot dispense drugs pursuant to a prescription for "office use."

III. Florida Board of Pharmacy (§ 465.004)
  A. Purpose
   1. The Florida Board of Pharmacy was established by the legislature to ensure that every pharmacist practicing in this state and every pharmacy meet minimum requirements for safe practice.
   2. The Florida Board of Pharmacy is responsible for the licensure, monitoring, and education of pharmacy professionals

to assure competency and safety to practice in their service to the people of Florida.

STUDY TIP: Remember, the purpose of the Board of Pharmacy is to protect the public health, safety, and welfare. The Board of Pharmacy is not responsible for advocating for pharmacists or pharmacies.

B. Organization
1. The Florida Board of Pharmacy is one of many regulatory boards under the Florida Department of Health. It is composed of 9 members.
2. Seven members must be licensed pharmacists who are residents of Florida and who have been engaged in the practice of pharmacy in Florida for at least 4 years. The other 2 members are consumer members.
3. The pharmacist members must include:
    a. At least 2 pharmacists practicing in a community pharmacy;
    b. At least 2 pharmacists practicing in an institutional pharmacy (Class II, Modified Class II, or Class III); and
    c. The remaining 3 pharmacists may be practicing in any practice setting.
4. The consumer members:
    a. Must be residents of Florida;
    b. May not have ever been licensed as a pharmacist;
    c. May not be connected with the pharmacy profession in any manner; and
    d. May not be connected in any manner with a drug manufacturer or wholesaler.
5. At least one member of the Board of Pharmacy (either pharmacist or consumer member) must be 60 years of age or older.

C. Appointment and Terms
1. Board of Pharmacy members are appointed by the Governor and confirmed by the Florida Senate.
2. Board members are appointed for 4-year terms; however, if a Board member's term ends, they may continue to serve until a new Board member has been appointed.
3. A Board member may not serve more than two full terms; however, if a member's term expires, they may remain on the Board until a new appointment is made by the Governor.

Note: The Board is run by an Executive Director. The Executive Director is an employee of the Department of Health. The Executive Director is not one of the 9 Board of Pharmacy members and does not have to be a pharmacist.

IV. Definitions

STUDY TIP: Definitions are often the key to understanding legal topics and answering legal questions. Always be sure to read the definition section of a statute or rule carefully. In addition, Florida statutory definitions sometimes contain definitions within definitions and sometimes place specific requirements on pharmacists and pharmacies directly in the definitions rather than in a separate section. For all these reasons, it is imperative to read and understand definitions. Some of the most important definitions from the Florida Pharmacy Act are provided below.

A. Consultant pharmacist—a pharmacist licensed by the department and certified as a consultant pharmacist pursuant to § 465.0125.

STUDY TIP: Florida law requires all institutional pharmacies (including hospitals) to be under the direction of a consultant pharmacist, and a consultant pharmacist license is a separate additional license from a pharmacist license with additional requirements. *See licensure section below.*

B. Dispense—the transfer of possession of one or more doses of a medicinal drug by a pharmacist to the ultimate consumer or her or his agent. As an element of dispensing, the pharmacist shall, prior to the actual physical transfer, interpret and assess the prescription order for potential adverse reactions, interactions, and dosage regimen she or he deems appropriate in the exercise of her or his professional judgment, and the pharmacist shall certify that the medicinal drug called for by the prescription is ready for transfer. The pharmacist shall also provide counseling on proper drug usage, either orally or in writing, if in the exercise of her or his professional judgment counseling is necessary. The actual sales transaction and delivery of such drug shall not be considered dispensing. The administration shall not be considered dispensing.

Note: This is an example of the Florida law placing mandatory requirements in the definition section of the law, which is a bit unusual. The intent is to make it clear that the acts of assessing a prescription for potential adverse reactions, interactions, and dosage regimen as well as patient counseling are considered part of the definition of dispense, but the use of the word "shall" in the definition makes the drug use review requirement mandatory. While the definition appears to make patient counseling mandatory, a careful reading indicates counseling is required only if the pharmacist deems it necessary. The specific requirements for drug use review and patient counseling, including the requirement for making an offer to counsel, are more detailed and can be found in Rules 64B16-27.810 and 64B16-27.820, respectively. See Chapter 4, Sections III.I.2. and 3

C. Medicinal drugs or "drugs"—means those substances or preparations commonly known as "prescription" or "legend" drugs, which are required by federal or state law to be dispensed only on a prescription but shall not include patents or proprietary preparations as hereafter defined.

D. Patent or proprietary preparation (OTC drugs)—a medicine in its unbroken, original package which is sold to the public by, or under the authority of, the manufacturer or primary distributor thereof and which is not misbranded under the provisions of the Florida Food, Drug and Cosmetic Act.

E. Pharmacy—includes a community pharmacy, an institutional pharmacy, a nuclear pharmacy, a special pharmacy, and an internet pharmacy.

   1. Community pharmacy—includes every location where medicinal drugs are compounded, dispensed, stored, or sold or where prescriptions are filled or dispensed on an outpatient basis.
   2. Institutional pharmacy—includes every location in a hospital, clinic, nursing home, dispensary, sanitarium, extended care facility, or other facility, hereinafter referred to as "healthcare institutions," where medicinal drugs are compounded, dispensed, stored, or sold.
   3. Nuclear pharmacy—includes every location where radioactive drugs and chemicals within the classification of medicinal drugs are compounded, dispensed, stored, or sold. The term "nuclear pharmacy" does not include hospitals licensed under Chapter 395 or the nuclear medicine facilities of such hospitals.

4. Special pharmacy—includes every location where medicinal drugs are compounded, dispensed, stored, or sold if such locations are not otherwise defined in this subsection.
5. Internet pharmacy—includes locations not otherwise licensed or issued a permit under this chapter, within or outside this state, which use the internet to communicate with or obtain information from consumers in this state and use such communication or information to fill or refill prescriptions or to dispense, distribute, or otherwise engage in the practice of pharmacy in this state.

The pharmacy department of any permittee shall be considered closed whenever a Florida licensed pharmacist is not present and on duty. The term "not present and on duty" shall not be construed to prevent a pharmacist from exiting the prescription department for the purposes of consulting or responding to inquiries or providing assistance to patients or customers, attending to personal hygiene needs, or performing any other function for which the pharmacist is responsible, provided that such activities are conducted in a manner consistent with the pharmacist's responsibility to provide pharmacy services.

Note: This provision is listed at the end of the definition of "pharmacy" and likely applies to all of the pharmacy permits listed above.

F. Practice of the profession of pharmacy—includes compounding, dispensing, and consulting concerning contents, therapeutic values, and uses of any medicinal drug; consulting concerning therapeutic values and interactions of patent or proprietary preparations, whether pursuant to prescriptions or in the absence and entirely independent of such prescriptions or orders; and conducting other pharmaceutical services. For purposes of this subsection, the term "other pharmaceutical services" means monitoring the patient's drug therapy and assisting the patient in the management of his or her drug therapy, and includes reviewing and making recommendations regarding the patient's drug therapy and healthcare status in communication with the patient's prescribing healthcare provider as licensed under Chapter 458 (Medical Doctors and some PAs and APRNs), Chapter 459 (Osteopathic Doctors and some PAs and APRNs), Chapter 461 (Podiatrists), or Chapter 466 (Dentists), or similar statutory provision in another jurisdiction, or such provider's agent or such other persons as specifically authorized by the patient, and initiating, modifying, or discontinuing drug therapy for a chronic health condition under a collaborative pharmacy practice agreement. This subsection may not be interpreted to permit an alteration of a prescriber's directions, the diagnosis or treatment of any disease, the initiation of any drug therapy, the practice of medicine, or the practice of osteopathic medicine unless otherwise permitted by law or specifically authorized by § 465.1865 (Collaborative Practice for Chronic Health Conditions) or § 465.1895 (testing or screening for and treatment of minor, nonchronic health conditions). The term "practice of the profession of pharmacy" also includes any other act, service, operation, research, or transaction incidental to, or forming a part of, any of the foregoing acts, requiring, involving, or employing the science or art of any branch of the pharmaceutical profession, study, or training, and shall expressly permit a pharmacist to transmit information from persons authorized to prescribe medicinal drugs to their patients. The practice of the profession of pharmacy also includes the administration of vaccines to adults pursuant to § 465.189, the testing or screening for and treatment of minor, nonchronic health conditions pursuant to § 465.1895, and the preparation of prepackaged drug products in facilities holding Class III institutional pharmacy permits. The term also includes the ordering and evaluating of any laboratory or clinical testing; conducting patient assessments; and modifying, discontinuing, or administering medicinal drugs pursuant to § 465.0125 by a consultant pharmacist.

Note: This definition likely inadvertently omitted communication with prescribing healthcare providers licensed under Chapter 474 (Veterinarians).

G. Prescription—includes any order for drugs or medicinal supplies written or transmitted by any means of communication by a duly licensed practitioner authorized by the laws of the state to prescribe such drugs or medicinal supplies and intended to be dispensed by a pharmacist. The term also includes an orally transmitted order by the lawfully designated agent of such practitioner. The term also includes an order written or transmitted by a practitioner licensed to practice in a jurisdiction other than this state, but only if the pharmacist called upon to dispense such order determines, in the exercise of her or his professional judgment, that the order is valid and necessary for the treatment of a chronic or recurrent illness. The term "prescription" also includes a pharmacist's order for a product selected from the formulary created pursuant to § 465.186. Prescriptions may be retained in written form or the pharmacist may cause them to be recorded in a data processing system, provided that such order can be produced in printed form upon lawful request.

V. Licensure of Individuals
   A. Licensure of Pharmacists
   1. Licensure by examination (§ 465.007)
      a. Complete application form and pay examination fee
      b. Must be at least 18 years of age
      c. Must be recipient of a degree from an accredited school or college of pharmacy; or have graduated from a school or college of pharmacy outside the United States and passed TOEFL, TSE, and FPGEE and have 500 hours of supervised work activity program. *See Rule 64B16-26.2031*
      d. Must submit proof of completion of internship program approved by the Board that shall not exceed 2,080 hours
   2. Additional Information on Licensure by Examination (Rules 64B16-26.200 and 64B16-203)
      a. Must pass North American Pharmacist Licensure Examination (NAPLEX) with a scaled score of 75 or higher
      b. Must pass Multistate Pharmacy Jurisprudence Examination (MPJE)—Florida Version with a score of 75 or greater.
      Note: The rule incorrectly states a passing score is 75%, but it is not actually a percentage score.
      c. All requirements for licensure must be met within one year of receipt of application or else have to be reapplied
      d. Successful examination scores may be used upon reapplication only if completed within 3 years of reapplication
   3. Licensure by endorsement (§ 465.0075)
      Note: Florida uses the term "endorsement," but this is similar to what is referred to as reciprocity in most states.
      a. Must meet age, internship, and education requirements in § 465.007
      b. Must have obtained a passing score on NAPLEX
      c. Must submit evidence of being licensed and actively practicing pharmacy in another jurisdiction for at least

2 of the immediately preceding 5 years, or submit evidence of successful completion of Board-approved postgraduate training or Board-approved clinical competency examination within the year preceding application, or have completed internship requirements within the preceding 2 years
  d. Must obtain a passing score on the MPJE—Florida Version
  e. Successful examination scores may be used upon reapplication only if completed within 3 years of reapplication
  f. If licensed in another state for more than 2 years, must submit proof of 30 hours of continuing education for the 2 years preceding application
  g. May not be under investigation in any jurisdiction
  h. May not have had a license suspended or revoked in another state or currently be subject to discipline in another state
 4. Renewal of Pharmacist License (§§ 465.008, 465.009)
  a. Must submit renewal application (renewal is done online), pay fee, and comply with continuing education requirements. *See details for continuing education requirements in B. below.*
  b. Licenses renew biennially (every 2 years) on September 30th of odd-number years
  c. Person licensed for 50 years or more is exempt from payment of renewal or delinquent fee and is given a lifetime license
B. Continuing Education (CE) Requirements (§ 465.009 and Rule 64B16-26.103(1))
 1. To renew a pharmacist license, a pharmacist must obtain 30 hours of continuing education in courses approved by the Board during the 24 months prior to expiration of the license.
 2. Pharmacists must complete 2 hours of a Board-approved course on medication errors. These hours may be part of the required 30 hours of CE.
 3. Pharmacists must complete 2 hours of Board-approved CE on Validation of Prescriptions for Controlled Substances as required in Rule 64B16-27.831. *See Chapter 2*

4. At least 10 hours must be from live seminars, video teleconferences, or interactive computer-based applications.
5. A pharmacist certified to administer vaccines or epinephrine auto-injectors must complete a 3-hour CE course on the safe and effective administration of vaccines and epinephrine auto-injection as part of the required 30 hours of CE.
6. Initial Renewal
    a. A 1 hour HIV/AIDS CE course is required as part of the initial renewal of a license.
    b. If you are renewing your license for the first time and your initial renewal occurs 12 months or more after initial licensure date, you are required to complete 15 hours of CE (of which 5 hours must be live), including 2 hours of medication errors, 2 hours of controlled substances, and 1 hour in HIV/AIDS.
    c. If your initial renewal occurs less than 12 months from your initial licensure date, you are required to complete 1 hour in HIV/AIDS, 2 hours of medication errors, and 2 hours of controlled substances.
7. Requirement for Instruction on Human Trafficking (Florida Statute § 546.0341)
    a. Legislation passed in 2019 required most healthcare professionals (including pharmacists) to complete a board-approved, 1-hour continuing education course on human trafficking by January 1, 2021. The course must address both sex trafficking and labor trafficking, how to identify individuals who may be victims of human trafficking, how to report cases of human trafficking, and resources available to victims.
    b. This was a onetime requirement and does not have to be completed with every two-year renewal.
    c. The law also requires posting a sign regarding human trafficking. *See Chapter 4, Section II. N.7.*
    Note: *The Board has not adopted any rules on this. Additional information can be found at* http://www.flhealthsource.gov/humantrafficking/
8. Methods of Obtaining CE
    a. All programs approved by the Accreditation Council for Pharmacy Education (ACPE) are deemed approved for general CE for pharmacists.

STUDY TIP: Do not get mixed up between continuing education hours and continuing education units. Nearly everyone tracks CE by hours, but ACPE tracks continuing education units or CEUs, which means a one-hour CE course will be accredited as 0.1 CEUs. If you see an ACPE course accredited for 0.3 CEUs, that equals 3 CE hours.

      b. Licensees may obtain 5 hours of CE in subject matter of Risk Management by attending one full day of a Board meeting at which disciplinary hearings are conducted. The maximum CE allowable by this method is 10 hours. *Note: You cannot receive CE for attendance at a Board meeting if you are required to appear before the Board.*
      c. Up to 5 hours of CE credit may be obtained by performing volunteer services to the indigent or to underserved populations or in areas of critical need within the state. One hour is awarded for every two hours of volunteer work.
      d. Completion of post-professional degree programs from accredited colleges or schools of pharmacy. Five hours of CE per semester hour may be claimed for courses completed during the renewal period.
      e. A volunteer expert witness providing expert witness opinions for cases being reviewed by the Department of Health shall receive 5 hours of CE in the subject matter of risk management. The maximum CE allowable by this method is 10 hours.
      f. The presenter of a live seminar, a live video teleconference, or through an interactive computer-based application may receive one credit for each course hour presented, but may not receive additional credit for presenting the same course on multiple occasions.
      g. A pharmacist who earns general CE in another state that is not ACPE approved but is approved by the Board of Pharmacy in the other state can apply that CE to the Florida CE requirements.

9. Tripartite Continuing Education Committee (Rules 64B16-26.600 and 64B16-26.601)
      a. Has authority to approve CE providers and approval of courses submitted by providers.
      b. Comprised of equal representation from the Board of Pharmacy, each College and School of Pharmacy in the state, and practicing pharmacists.

- c. The Tripartite Committee approves CE courses from approved providers or individuals who are non-approved providers for general CE courses and also specific Florida CE that may be required, such as:
  - (1) Initial Consultant Pharmacist Certification
  - (2) Consultant Pharmacist Recertification
  - (3) Nuclear Pharmacist Recertification
  - (4) Medication Errors
  - (5) HIV/AIDS
  - (6) Laboratory Tests
  - (7) Laws and Rules (required Board-ordered CE in disciplinary cases)
  - (8) Quality Related Events
  - (9) Validation of Prescriptions or Controlled Substances
- d. The Tripartite Committee uses standards for approval of CE Courses found in Rule 64B16-26.60.

10. Board-Ordered Disciplinary Continuing Education Courses (Rule 64B16-26.6012)
    - a. CE Courses being taken as part of a disciplinary order, unless otherwise ordered by the Board, may be conducted by any method, including live, correspondence, or distance education.
    - b. CE Courses on Laws and Rules shall be at least 12 hours in length and must cover specific topics as outlined in the rule.
    - c. CE Courses on Quality Related Events shall be at least 8 hours in length and cover specific topics as outlined in the rule.
      Note: This type of CE is often required after a dispensing error.
11. Tracking Continuing Education
    - a. All healthcare providers licensed by the Florida Department of Health, including pharmacists, must use an electronic system called CE Broker for tracking their continuing education. A basic account with CE Broker is free.
    - b. Florida-approved CE providers will automatically report your hours to CE Broker, but you may have to manually report hours from national providers such as ACPE courses.

- **c.** NABP also has an online CE tracking service called CPE Monitor, and all ACPE-approved providers report CE hours to CPE Monitor.
- **d.** The Florida Department of Health will not allow you to renew your license if you do not have the required CE hours reported in CE Broker.

C. Consultant Pharmacist License (§ 465.0125 and Rules 64B16-26.300, 64B16-26.301, 64B16-26.302, and 64B16-26.320)

1. A Consultant Pharmacist License is an additional license that a pharmacist may obtain and is required for a pharmacist to serve as the Consultant Pharmacist of Record for an Institutional Pharmacy permit.
2. Requirements:
   - **a.** Must hold a license as a pharmacist which is active and in good standing.
   - **b.** Must successfully complete a consultant pharmacist course of no fewer than 12 hours sponsored by an accredited college of pharmacy and approved by the Tripartite Committee.
     Note: At the time of publication of this book, the Board had proposed changes to Rule 64B16-26.300 to require the initial consultant pharmacist course be 20 hours.
   - **c.** The consultant pharmacist course must cover the subject matter in Rule 64B16-26.300 and must include a cognitive test that the applicant must pass. See detail in rule, but major topics include:
     - (1) Jurisprudence (laws and regulations)
     - (2) Policies and procedures
     - (3) Administrative responsibilities
     - (4) Professional responsibilities
     - (5) The institutional environment
     - (6) Nuclear pharmacy
   - **d.** Successfully completing a period of assessment and evaluation under the supervision of a preceptor within one year of completion of the consultant pharmacist course. This must be completed over no more than 3 consecutive months and shall include at least 40 hours of training in specific areas. *See rule details for specific areas.*
     Note: At the time of publication of this book, the Board had proposed, but not finalized, changes to Rule 64B16-26.300 to eliminate this requirement.

- e. In order to serve as a consultant pharmacist preceptor, a person must be a consultant pharmacist of record at an institutional pharmacy, have at least one year of experience as a consultant pharmacist of record, and not serve as a preceptor to more than 2 applicants at one time.
3. Collaborative Practice by Consultant Pharmacists
   - a. A consultant pharmacist may provide medication management services in a healthcare facility within the framework of a written collaborative practice agreement between the pharmacist and a healthcare facility medical director or a physician, a podiatric physician, or a dentist.
   - b. A consultant pharmacist may only provide medication management services, conduct patient assessments, and order and evaluate laboratory or clinical testing for patients of the healthcare practitioner with whom the consultant pharmacist has a written collaborative practice agreement.
   - c. A written collaborative practice agreement must outline the circumstances under which the consultant pharmacist may:
     - (1) Order and evaluate any laboratory or clinical tests to promote and evaluate patient health and wellnesss and monitor drug therapy and treatment outcomes.
     - (2) Conduct patient assessments as appropriate to evaluate and monitor drug therapy.
     - (3) Modify or discontinue medicinal drugs as outlined in the agreed-upon patient-specific order or preapproved treatment protocol under the direction of a physician. However, a consultant pharmacist may not modify or discontinue medicinal drugs prescribed by a healthcare practitioner who does not have a written collaborative practice agreement with the consultant pharmacist.
     - (4) Administer medicinal drugs.
   - d. Consultant pharmacists who wish to order and evaluate laboratory tests under § 465.0125 must complete a 3-hour initial certification course meeting the requirements of Rule 64B16-26.320. This 3-hour certification course may apply to the 24 hours of consultant pharmacist CE required to renew a consultant pharmacist license.

4. Renewal of Consultant Pharmacist License
   a. A consultant pharmacist must complete 24 hours of consultant pharmacist CE that meets the requirements of Board Rule 64B16-26.302. *See rule for details*
   b. The 24 hours of CE required for consultant pharmacist recertification *may not* be used toward the general 30-hour CE requirements for a pharmacist license.

STUDY TIP: You should be familiar with the consultant pharmacist licensure requirements, as these requirements are unique to Florida.

---

   c. Consultant pharmacists that wish to continue to order and evaluate laboratory tests must complete at least one hour of CE on ordering and evaluating laboratory tests in order to renew their license. This one hour may apply to the 24 hours of consultant pharmacist CE required to renew a consultant pharmacist license.
D. Registration of Pharmacy Interns (§ 465.013 and Rules 64B16-26.2032, 64B16-26.2033, and 64B16-26.400)
   1. Pharmacist interns in the state must be registered before being employed.
   2. Intern must be enrolled in an internship program at an accredited college or school of pharmacy or have graduated from one and not yet be licensed in the state.
   3. An intern may not perform any acts relating to the filling, compounding, or dispensing of medicinal drugs unless it is done under the direct and immediate personal supervision of a licensed pharmacist.
   4. Within 30 days of termination in enrollment in an intern program, or withdrawal of registration or attendance in an accredited school or college of pharmacy, all registered interns shall report such change in enrollment, registration, or attendance to the Board.
   5. Foreign pharmacy graduate interns must be supervised at a ratio of one pharmacist to one intern.
   6. Pharmacists serving as preceptors of pharmacy interns:
      a. Shall accept responsibility for professional guidance and training of the intern and be able to devote time to preceptor training sessions and instruction of the intern;
      b. Must hold current licensure in the state in which pharmacy is practiced;

      c. May not have a license revoked, suspended, on probation, or subject to payment of an unpaid fine, or be subject of ongoing disciplinary proceedings; and
      d. Must agree to assist the college or school of pharmacy in achievement of the educational objectives, and provide documentation of the pharmacist's continued professional education and of active involvement in a patient-centered practice.
   7. A total of 2,080 hours of internship are required to be licensed as a pharmacist.
      a. All internship hours may be obtained prior to the applicant's graduation.
      b. Hours worked in excess of 50 hours per week prior to an applicant's graduation, or in excess of 60 hours per week after an applicant's graduation, will not be credited.
E. Registration of Pharmacy Technicians (§ 465.014 Rules 64B16-26.103(4), 64B16-26.350, and 64B16-26.351)
   1. Any person wishing to work as a pharmacy technician in Florida must register with the Board by filing an application and pay a registration fee.
   2. An applicant must be at least 17 years of age.
   3. Applicants must have completed a pharmacy technician training program approved by the Board. Approved programs include:
      a. Preapproved pharmacy technician training programs;
      b. Federal Armed Services programs;
      c. Other non-employer-based programs; and
      d. Employer-sponsored training programs;
      See Board Rule 64B16-26.351 or the Board's website for details on approved training programs

STUDY TIP: Programs such as those offered by the Pharmacy Technician Certification Board (PTCB) or National Healthcareer Association (NHA), which both provide a Certified Pharmacy Technician examination and certification (CPhT), are not approved training programs. A certified pharmacy technician cannot practice in Florida until they are registered by the Board, which requires completing a pharmacy technician training program approved by the Board.

   4. A person whose license to practice pharmacy has been denied, suspended, or restricted for disciplinary reasons may not register as a pharmacy technician.

5. A pharmacy technician student who is enrolled in a pharmacy technician training program that is approved by the Board may be in a pharmacy to obtain practical training.
6. A pharmacy intern may be employed as a pharmacy technician without paying a registration fee or filing an application as a pharmacy technician.
7. Renewal of Registration
    a. Pharmacy technicians must complete no less than 20 hours of Board-approved CE in order to renew a registration.
    b. Pharmacy technicians must complete a 2-hour Board-approved course on medication errors. These hours may be part of the required 20 hours of CE.
    c. At least 4 hours of the 20 hours must be obtained at a live seminar, live video teleconference, or through an interactive computer-based application.
    d. Upon first renewal, pharmacy technicians must complete one contact hour of a Board-approved course on HIV/AIDS.
    e. Legislation passed in 2019 required most healthcare licensees, including pharmacy technicians, to complete a Board-approved, 1-hour continuing education course on human trafficking by January 1, 2021.
    f. All programs approved by the Accreditation Council for Pharmacy Education (ACPE) are deemed approved for general CE for pharmacy technicians.
    g. Pharmacy technicians may obtain 5 hours of CE in subject matter of Risk Management by attending one full day of a Board meeting at which disciplinary hearings are conducted. The maximum CE allowable by this method is 10 hours.
        Note: You cannot receive CE for attendance at a Board meeting if you are required to appear before the Board.

F. Additional License Rules for Individuals
    1. Nuclear Pharmacist License—*See Nuclear Pharmacies and Pharmacists in Chapter 4, Section V*
    2. Delinquent License and Reactivation (Rule 64B16-26.1021)
        Note: This rule applies to pharmacist licenses, consultant pharmacist licenses, nuclear pharmacist licenses, and pharmacy technician registrations.
        a. A license or registration that is not renewed in time automatically reverts to delinquent status.

    b. A licensee or registrant may request reinstatement of a delinquent license if all continuing education requirements are met and a reactivation fee is paid, but it must be done prior to the next renewal; i.e., within 2 years since license became delinquent.

STUDY TIP: Notice a delinquent license may only be reactivated within 2 years; after that, the license is void.

  3. Inactive Status and Reactivation (Rule 64B16-26.1004)
Note: This rule applies to pharmacist licenses, consultant pharmacist licenses, nuclear pharmacist licenses, and pharmacy technician registrations.
    a. Licensees may request to be placed on inactive status at time of renewal but must still pay an inactive license renewal fee.
    b. License can be reactivated by meeting required continuing education hours and paying a reactivation fee.

STUDY TIP: You cannot practice when your license is inactive. You also still have to pay a renewal fee. Unlike a delinquent license, you can keep a license inactive for more than 2 years as long as you continue to pay the renewal fee.

  4. Retired License Election (Rule 64B16-26.1005)
Note: This rule does not mention pharmacy technician registrations, so it appears to only apply to pharmacists' licenses.
    a. A licensee may elect to place their license on retired status by making a request to the Board and paying a retired status fee and an unlicensed activity fee.
    b. Before reactivating a retired license, the licensee must meet all continuing education requirements for all 2-year periods when the license was retired.
    c. If a pharmacist has been on retired status for 5 years or more, they must:
      (1) pass the MPJE for Florida if they have been actively practicing for at least part of those 5 years in another jurisdiction; or
      (2) pass both the MPJE and NAPLEX if they not been actively practicing in another jurisdiction for 5 or more years.

5. Exemptions for Members of the Armed Forces and Spouses (Rule 64B16-26.104)
   a. Any pharmacist or pharmacy technician on active duty with the Armed Forces of the United States who at the time of becoming a member of the Armed Forces was in good standing with the Board is exempt from all license renewal provisions so long as the licensee is on active duty and for 6 months after discharge.
   b. A pharmacist or pharmacy technician who is a spouse of a member of the Armed Forces of the United States and was caused to be absent from the State of Florida because of the spouse's duties shall be exempt from all license renewal provisions.
   Note: This apparently includes renewing licenses or registrations, meeting continuing education requirements, and paying renewal fees.
6. Proof of License; Display of License (Rule 64B16-27.100)
   a. Every pharmacist, pharmacy intern, and registered pharmacy technician must maintain proof of current licensure that is readily retrievable upon request by any representative of the Department of Health or the Board or any member of the public.
   b. A pharmacy may display the license of each pharmacy employee or alternatively may display a notice that licenses are available for viewing upon request.
   c. Every pharmacist, pharmacy intern, or registered pharmacy technician must be identified by means of an identification badge.

VI. Pharmacy Permits
A. General Permit Requirements (§ 465.022 and Rules 64B16-28.100(1) and (2) and 64B16-28.2021)
   1. Before engaging in the operation of a pharmacy, a person or business entity must file a sworn application, which may include a set of fingerprints from each person having an ownership interest of 5% or greater and include any person who, directly or indirectly, manages, oversees, or controls the operation of the applicant, including officers and members of the Board of Directors if a corporation.
   2. For corporations having more than $100 million of business taxable assets in the state, only the prescription department

manager or consultant pharmacist of record is required to submit fingerprints.
3. An application for a pharmacy permit must include written policies and procedures for preventing controlled substance dispensing based on fraudulent representations or invalid practitioner-patient relationships.
4. Passing an on-site inspection is required before the issuance of a new pharmacy permit, for a change of ownership, a change of address, or a change of location.
5. A pharmacy permit is only valid for a specific entity under a specific name and single physical location listed on the permit. The name must be the name in which the company is doing business and appear on purchase and sales invoices.
6. A single physical location is generally an address, but it may cover a broader area as long as it is a contiguous area under the control of the permit holder. Such an area cannot be more than ½ mile from the central location of the permit.

STUDY TIP: This is similar to a campus registration for DEA. Pharmacists at large facilities should ensure that both their state and permit and DEA registration cover the entire campus.

7. A pharmacy permit is not transferable. Upon the sale of a pharmacy, a new application must be filed and a new permit obtained. *See Rule 64B16-28.2021 for change of ownership rules*

B. Community Pharmacy Permits (§ 465.018 and Rule 64B16-28.100(2))
1. A community pharmacy permit is required for every location where medicinal drugs are compounded, dispensed, stored, or sold or where prescriptions are filled or dispensed on an outpatient basis.
2. A community pharmacy permit may not be issued unless a licensed pharmacist is designated as the prescription department manager. *See Chapter 4, Section III. A. for details*

STUDY TIP: Florida uses the term "prescription department manager" for community pharmacies to identify the pharmacist who is responsible for the legal operation of the pharmacy. This person is often referred to as a "pharmacist-in-charge" or "PIC" in other states.

C. Institutional Pharmacy Permits (§ 465.019 and Rules 64B16-28100(3) and 64B16-28.501(1))
   1. General
      a. An institutional pharmacy permit is required for any location in any healthcare institution where medicinal drugs are compounded, dispensed, stored, or sold.
      b. An institutional pharmacy permit may not be issued unless a licensed pharmacist is designated as the consultant pharmacist of record.
      c. Institutional pharmacies may not dispense drugs to outpatients unless they obtain a community pharmacy permit. *Note: Class II and III Institutional Pharmacies may do limited outpatient dispensing with a Special—Limited Community Pharmacy Permit. Also, see Chapter 4 for a limited exception for emergency rooms.*
   2. Class I Institutional Pharmacy Permit
      a. This permit is for institutional pharmacies in which all medicinal drugs are administered from individual prescription containers to the individual patient and in which medicinal drugs are not dispensed on the premises, except that these facilities may purchase medical oxygen for administration to residents.
      b. No medicinal drugs may be dispensed in a Class I institutional pharmacy.

STUDY TIP: This permit is generally for nursing homes and Intermediate Care Facilities for Developmentally Disabled persons (ICF/DD). Notice that no drugs are dispensed at a Class I Institutional Pharmacy. This is because the drugs are dispensed by the pharmacy servicing the facility. Florida is fairly unique in that it requires a pharmacy permit at these types of facilities even though no drugs are being dispensed at the location.

   3. Class II Institutional Pharmacy Permit
      This permit is for institutional pharmacies that employ the services of a registered pharmacist or pharmacists who, in practicing institutional pharmacy, shall provide dispensing and consulting services *on the premises* to patients of that institution, for use on the premises of that institution.

STUDY TIP: This permit is generally for hospitals.

4. Modified Class II Institutional Pharmacy Permit
   a. This permit is for institutional pharmacies in short-term, primary care treatment centers that meet all the requirements for a Class II permit, except space and equipment requirements.

STUDY TIP: Modified Class II pharmacies typically do not have a full-time pharmacist on duty, and drugs are administered to patients on the premises. No outpatient dispensing is permitted.

   b. Examples of facilities that would have this permit include primary alcoholism treatment centers, free-standing emergency rooms, rapid in/out surgical centers, certain county health programs, and certain correctional institutions.
   c. All Modified Class II institutional pharmacies must have a consultant pharmacist who provides on-site consultations at least once per month.
   d. All Modified Class II pharmacies shall have a policy and procedure manual with specific required information, including definitive information on drugs and strengths to be stocked. *See Rule 64B16-28.702(4)(5) and (6) for details*
   e. Modified Class II pharmacies may contract with a Special Parenteral/Enteral Extended Scope Pharmacy for services.
   f. Modified Class II pharmacies must have a Pharmacy Services Committee that meets at least annually.
   g. There are several subcategories of Modified Class II permits.
      (1) Type A—Has a formulary of not more than 15 medicinal drugs (excluding drugs in an emergency kit) and in which the medicinal drugs are stored in bulk. Controlled substances may not exceed 100 dosage units unless an exception is granted by the Board of Pharmacy. An example would be an alcoholism treatment center.
      (2) Type B—Has an expanded formulary and in which medicinal drugs are stored in bulk and patient-specific form. Examples include urgent care centers,

outpatient surgery centers, and correctional institutions.
- (3) Type C—Has an expanded formulary and medicinal drugs are stored in patient-specific form. No bulk drugs are allowed. An example would be a jail with a small inmate population. Drugs are self-administered under supervision.
5. Class III Institutional Pharmacy Permit
   a. This permit is for institutional pharmacies, including central distribution facilities, affiliated with a hospital, that provide the same services authorized by a Class II institutional pharmacy.
   b. This permit allows the pharmacy to:
      (1) Dispense, distribute, compound, and fill prescriptions for medicinal drugs;
      Note: Both Class II and Class III Institutional may only do limited outpatient dispensing and must obtain a Special—Limited Community Pharmacy Permit to do so.
      (2) Prepare prepackaged drug products; and
      (3) Conduct other pharmaceutical services for the affiliated hospital and for entities under common control that each are permitted to possess medicinal drugs.
   c. A facility may have only a Class III permit or may hold a Class III permit in conjunction with other pharmacy permits.
   Note: Prior to the establishment of this permit, hospital pharmacies that prepackaged drugs or provided centralized distribution for affiliated locations, and hospitals that participated in the 340(b) drug discount program and arranged for a wholesale distributor to ship drugs to a contract pharmacy, had to obtain a restricted drug distribution permit from the Florida Department of Professional Regulation. The Class III Institutional permit exempts hospitals from having to do that.
D. Special Pharmacy Permits (§ 465.0196 and Rules 64B16-28.100(5) and 64B16-28.800)
   1. Special Pharmacy Permits are required for any location where medicinal drugs are compounded, dispensed, stored, or sold but is not a community pharmacy, institutional pharmacy, nuclear pharmacy, or internet pharmacy. These

pharmacies provide miscellaneous specialized pharmacy services.
2. A permit will not be issued unless a special pharmacy has a licensed pharmacist designated to undertake professional supervision of the compounding and dispensing of all drugs.
3. An applicant for any special pharmacy permit must provide the Board of Pharmacy with a policy and procedure manual that sets forth a detailed description of the type of pharmacy services to be provided.
4. The Board has designated 8 specific types of Special Pharmacy Permits by rule as follows:
   a. Special Limited Community Permit (Rule 64B16-28.810)—required for any Institutional Class II (hospital) pharmacy that dispenses to employees, medical staff, and their dependents; patients of the emergency room; and discharged patients of the hospital, not to exceed a 3-day supply.
   Note: There is an exception to the 3-day supply limit for products that come in multi-dose packages, such as inhalers, ocular products, otic products, insulin vials or pens, bulk antibiotic suspensions, topical agents, and methylprednisolone dose packages.
   b. Special Sterile Products and Special Parenteral/Enteral Compounding (Rule 64B28.820)—required for any pharmacy that provides parenteral (IV), enteral, and cytotoxic pharmacy services to outpatients.
      (1) This may be a stand-alone permit or be used in conjunction with a Community Pharmacy Permit or Special Closed System Pharmacy Permit;
      (2) Required to have a Prescription Department Manager;
      (3) Required to maintain a patient profile;
      (4) Required to have a policy and procedure manual including a quality assurance program;
      (5) Must meet specific requirements for space and all compounding requirements.
   c. Special Parenteral/Enteral Extended Scope Permit Rule (64B16-28.860)—required for pharmacies to compound and dispense patient-specific parenteral/enteral drugs in conjunction with an institutional permit.
   Note: This permit allows a pharmacy to prepare patient-specific sterile products for patients in a hospital or other

institutional facility. It can also be used by a hospital to operate a home infusion/enteral service.

- d. Special Sterile Compounding Permit (SSCP) (Rule 64B16-28.802)—required for any pharmacy or outsourcing facility compounding sterile products.
    - (1) An SSCP is required for all outsourcing facilities. If the outsourcing facility also engages in patient-specific compounding, it must also have either a community pharmacy permit or institutional permit depending on the type of practice engaged in.
    - (2) An SSCP is an additional permit for pharmacies compounding sterile products.
    - (3) An SSCP is not required for a Special Parenteral/Enteral or Special Parenteral/Enteral Extended Scope pharmacy if that pharmacy holds no other pharmacy permit and is not registered as an outsourcing facility.
    - (4) An SSCP is not required for a Modified Type B Class II Institutional Pharmacy if the pharmacy only compounds low-risk-level sterile products for immediate use.
- e. Special Closed System Pharmacy Permit (Rule 64B16-28.830)—required for any pharmacy that dispenses to facilities where prescriptions are individually prepared for the ultimate consumer, including nursing homes, jails, Adult Congregate Living Facilities, Intermediate Care Facilities for Individuals with Intellectual Disabilities (ICF-IIDs), or other custodial care facilities. Must have 24-hour on-call service.
- f. Special ESRD (End Stage Renal Disease) Permit (Rule 64B16-28.850)—provides dialysis products and supplies to persons with chronic kidney failure for self-administration at the person's home or specified address.
- g. Special ALF Permit (Rule 64B16-28.870)—an optional license for Assisted Living Facilities using drugs in unit-dose packaging. Drugs may not be dispensed on the premises. Allows medicinal drugs (not controlled substances) to be returned to the dispensing pharmacy under Rule 64B16-28.118.
- h. Special Internet Pharmacy Permit Rule (64B16-28.100(6) and § 465.0197)—required for any location not otherwise

issued a permit, within or outside the state, that uses the sinternet to communicate with or obtain information from consumers and uses this information to fill or refill prescriptions or to dispense, distribute, or otherwise engage in the practice of pharmacy in Florida.

E. Other Permits
  1. Nuclear Pharmacy Permit—*See Nuclear Pharmacies and Pharmacists in Chapter 4, Section V*
  2. Nonresident Pharmacy Permit (§ 465.0156 and Rules 64B16-32.001 and 64B16-32.005)
  a. Required for pharmacies located outside of Florida that ship, mail, or deliver, in any manner, a dispensed medicinal drug into Florida.
  b. Does not allow shipping, mailing, delivering, or dispensing a compounded sterile product into Florida.
  c. A nonresident pharmacy does not have to obtain a permit if it limits dispensing to one time per calendar year in an isolated transaction, which is defined as to a single, identifiable patient in Florida.
  3. Nonresident Sterile Compounding Permit (Rules 64B16-32.007 and 64B16-28.32.015)
  a. Required for pharmacies located outside of Florida that ship, mail, deliver, or dispense, in any manner, a patient-specific compounded sterile product into Florida.
  b. All applicants must have a current and satisfactory inspection report.
  4. Nonresident Sterile Compounding Outsourcing Facility Permit (Rule 64B16-32.009)
  a. Required for outsourcing facilities located outside of Florida to ship, mail, or deliver a sterile compounded product into Florida for office use.
  b. May also ship, mail, deliver, or dispense a patient-specific compounded sterile product into Florida.
  5. Animal Control Shelter Permit
  a. This permit is actually a Modified Class II Institutional permit, but for this permit a consultant pharmacist is not required.
  b. Must have a DEA registration.
  c. May only stock sodium pentobarbital and sodium pentobarbital with lidocaine, tiletamine hydrochloride, alone or combined with zolazepam, zylazine, ketamine,

acepromazine maleate, acetylpromazine, alone or combined with etorphine, and yohimbine hydrochloride, alone or combined with atipamezole, for euthanization or chemical immobilization of animals within their lawful possession.

Note: With the exception of sodium pentobarbital, sodium pentobarbital with lidocaine, and ketamine, these other drugs are veterinary drugs.

6. International Pharmacy Permit
   a. Pending federal approval, Florida will establish two programs to safely import FDA-approved prescription drugs into Florida:
      (1) The Canadian Drug Importation Program; and
      (2) The International Drug Importation Program.
   b. The Florida Board of Pharmacy is responsible for the creation and inspection of a new permit for an international export pharmacy.
   c. The law creates eligibility criteria for the types of prescription drugs to be imported, the importation process, safety standards, distribution requirements, and penalties for violations of the established program.
   d. Federal approval is required before the program may begin.
   e. The Department of Business and Professional Regulation is responsible for creating the international prescription drug importation program; the permits for pharmacy wholesalers and distributors; registration of drugs and devices; and operation of a pilot program upon authorization granted under federal law, rule, or approval.

VII. Florida Food Drug and Cosmetic Act—Chapter 499
A. Introduction
   1. The Florida Food Drug & Cosmetic Act (FFDCA) is similar to the Federal Food, Drug & Cosmetic Act discussed in Chapter 1.
   2. The FFDCA is enforced by the Florida Department of Business and Professional Regulation (DBPR) and not the Board of Pharmacy. DBPR's goal is to administer and enforce the FFDCA to prevent fraud, adulteration, misbranding, or false advertising in the preparation, manufacture, repackaging, or distribution of drugs, devices, and cosmetics.

3. Aside from the device and cosmetic sections, the FFDCA applies primarily to drug manufacturers, drug repackagers, drug wholesalers, medical gas/oxygen manufacturers and distributors, and others involved in the distribution (not dispensing) of drugs.
4. This review will focus on those sections of the FFDCA that impact pharmacy practice or may be included in the MPJE competency statements.

B. Selected Permits
1. Retail Pharmacy Wholesale Distributor
   a. Required for a retail (community) pharmacy that engages in wholesale distribution of prescription drugs.
   b. The wholesale distribution activity does not exceed 30% of the total annual purchases of prescription drugs.
   c. If the wholesale distribution activity exceeds the 30% maximum, the pharmacy must obtain a prescription drug wholesale distributor permit.
   d. The transfer (i.e., distribution) must be between a retail pharmacy and another retail pharmacy, or a Modified Class II institutional pharmacy, or a healthcare practitioner licensed in this state and authorized by law to dispense or prescribe prescription drugs.
2. Complimentary Drug Distributor
   a. This permit is required for any person that engages in the distribution of a complimentary drug (i.e., prescription drug samples).
   b. The FFDCA requirements for prescription drug samples are similar to the federal requirements under the PDMA.
   c. All expired prescription drug samples must be returned to the manufacturer or distributor who provided the sample.
3. Medical Oxygen Retailer
   a. This permit is required for an entity that is located in Florida and that sells or delivers medical oxygen directly to patients in Florida.
   b. The sale and delivery must be based on a prescription or an order from a practitioner authorized by law to prescribe.
   c. A pharmacy licensed under Chapter 465 does not require a permit as a medical oxygen retail establishment.

    d. A medical oxygen retail establishment may not possess, purchase, sell, or trade a medical gas other than medical oxygen.

STUDY TIP: This is one of the few examples where a prescription drug may be dispensed by an entity other than a pharmacy.

4. Veterinary Prescription Drug Retailer
    a. This permit is required for any person that sells veterinary prescription drugs to the public but does not include a pharmacy licensed under Chapter 465.
    b. The sale to the public must be based on a valid written order from a veterinarian licensed in Florida who has a valid client-veterinarian relationship with the purchaser's animal.
    c. Veterinary prescription drugs may not be sold in excess of the amount clearly indicated on the order or beyond the date indicated on the order.
    d. An order may not be valid for more than 1 year.
    e. A veterinary prescription drug retail establishment may not purchase, sell, trade, or possess human prescription drugs or any controlled substance. *Note: This does not say a veterinarian cannot prescribe a human prescription drug or wholesaler. It says a veterinarian's office that has this permit and dispenses veterinary drugs may not store or sell those drugs.*
    f. A veterinary prescription drug retail establishment must sell a veterinary prescription drug in the original, sealed manufacturer's container with all labeling intact and legible. The department may adopt by rule additional labeling requirements for the sale of a veterinary prescription drug.

STUDY TIP: This is an additional establishment that may dispense drugs but that is not a pharmacy.

5. Healthcare Clinic Establishment Registration
    a. This permit is required for the purchase of a prescription drug by a place of business at one general physical location that provides healthcare or veterinary services, which is owned and operated by a business entity

that has been issued a federal employer tax identification number.
- **b.** An individual practitioner who has the authority to prescribe drugs may generally purchase prescription drugs under their own license to be used in their office, but this permit allows a business, such as a clinic, to purchase prescription drugs that may be used by multiple providers at the clinic.
- **c.** A healthcare clinic establishment must have a qualifying practitioner who is responsible for complying with all legal and regulatory requirements related to the purchase, recordkeeping, storage, and handling of the prescription drugs. In addition, the qualifying practitioner shall be the practitioner whose name, establishment address, and license number is used on all distribution documents for prescription drugs purchased or returned by the healthcare clinic establishment.

C. Selected Violations
1. Adulteration and Misbranding of a Drug
   Note: The adulteration and misbranding provisions under the FFDCA are substantially similar to those under the federal rules as discussed in Chapter 1.
2. The refusal or constructive refusal to allow the DBPR to:
   - **a.** enter or inspect an establishment in which drugs, devices, or cosmetics are manufactured, processed, repackaged, sold, brokered, or held;
   - **b.** inspect any record of that establishment;
   - **c.** enter and inspect any vehicle that is being used to transport drugs, devices, or cosmetics; or
   - **d.** take samples of any drug, device, or cosmetic.
3. The purchase or receipt of a prescription drug from a person that is not authorized to distribute prescription drugs to that purchaser or recipient.
4. The sale or transfer of a prescription drug to a person that is not authorized under the law of the jurisdiction in which the person receives the drug to purchase or possess prescription drugs from the person selling or transferring the prescription drug.
5. Obtaining or attempting to obtain a prescription drug or device by fraud, deceit, misrepresentation, or subterfuge, or

engaging in misrepresentation or fraud in the distribution of a drug or device.
6. Charging a dispensing fee for dispensing, administering, or distributing a prescription drug sample.
7. Removing a pharmacy's dispensing label from a dispensed prescription drug with the intent to further distribute the prescription drug.
8. Distributing a prescription drug that was previously dispensed by a licensed pharmacy, unless such distribution is authorized in the Florida Pharmacy Act or rules.
9. Failure to acquire or deliver a transaction history, transaction information, or transaction statement as required.

D. Cancer Drug Donation Program
1. This program was established to facilitate the donation of cancer drugs and supplies to eligible patients.
2. Cancer drugs include drugs to treat cancer and its side effects but does not include any controlled substances.
3. A "donor" may be:
   a. A patient or patient representative who donates cancer drugs or supplies needed to administer cancer drugs that have been maintained within a closed drug delivery system;
   b. Healthcare facilities, nursing homes, hospices, or hospitals with closed drug delivery systems;
   c. Pharmacies, drug manufacturers, medical device manufacturers or suppliers, or wholesalers of drugs or supplies; or
   d. A physician who receives cancer drugs or supplies directly from a drug manufacturer, wholesale distributor, or pharmacy.
4. Institutional Class II (hospital) pharmacies can elect to participate in the program as a "participant facility" and accept donated cancer drugs and supplies under the rules adopted by the department for the program.
5. A cancer drug may only be accepted or dispensed under the program if the drug is in its original, unopened, sealed container, or in a tamper-evident unit-dose packaging, except that a cancer drug packaged in single-unit doses may be accepted and dispensed if the outside packaging is opened but the single-unit-dose packaging is unopened with tamper-resistant packaging intact.

6. A cancer drug may not be accepted or dispensed under the program if the drug bears an expiration date that is less than 6 months after the date the drug was donated or if the drug appears to have been tampered with or mislabeled as described in 7. below.
7. Prior to being dispensed to an eligible patient, the cancer drug or supplies donated under the program shall be inspected by a pharmacist to determine that the drug and supplies do not appear to have been tampered with or mislabeled.
8. A dispenser of donated cancer drugs or supplies may not submit a claim or otherwise seek reimbursement from any public or private third-party payor for donated cancer drugs or supplies dispensed to any patient under the program.
9. A donation of cancer drugs or supplies shall be made only at a participant facility. A participant facility may decline to accept a donation. A participant facility that accepts donated cancer drugs or supplies under the program shall comply with all applicable provisions of state and federal law relating to the storage and dispensing of the donated cancer drugs or supplies.
10. A participant facility that voluntarily takes part in the program may charge a handling fee sufficient to cover the cost of preparation and dispensing of cancer drugs or supplies under the program. The fee shall be established in rules adopted by the department.

CHAPTER FOUR
Florida Pharmacy Law—Part 2
Pharmacy Personnel and
Pharmacy Practice

CHAPTER FOUR
Florida Pharmacy Law—Part 2
Pharmacy Personnel and Pharmacy Practice

I. **Laws and Rules Applicable to Individuals**
   A. Pharmacists
      1. Practice of Pharmacy (Rule 64B16-27.1001)
         This rule sets forth the functions that only a pharmacist or registered intern acting under the direct and immediate personal supervision of a pharmacist may perform:
         a. Supervising and being responsible for the controlled substance inventory;
         b. Receiving verbal prescriptions;
         c. Interpreting and identifying prescription contents;
         d. Engaging in consultation with a practitioner regarding interpretation of a prescription and date in a patient profile;
            Note: The rule says "date," but this is likely a typo and was meant to be "data."
         e. Engaging in professional communication with practitioners, nurses, or other health professionals;
         f. Advising or consulting with a patient, both as to prescriptions and the patient profile record;
         g. Making the final check of a completed prescription, thereby assuming the complete responsibility for its preparation and accuracy;

STUDY TIP: Although this is listed in the rule that includes interns, this provision states that only a pharmacist may perform the final check of a prescription, so this is not something an intern can do. Only a pharmacist can make the final check of a completed prescription.

---

         h. Being personally available to the patient or the patient's agent for consultation; and
         i. When preparing parenteral and bulk solutions:
            (1) Interpreting and identifying all incoming orders; and
            (2) Being physically present and giving direction to registered pharmacy technicians for the reconstitution, addition of additives, or bulk compounding.

2. **Delegable and Non-Delegable Duties Rule (64B16-27.420)**
   This rule sets forth the tasks that may and may not be delegated to pharmacy technicians. The non-delegable tasks are therefore functions that only a pharmacist may perform. These include:
   a. receiving new, non-written (i.e., verbal) prescriptions or receiving any change in the medication, strength, or directions of an existing prescription;
      Note: This point is made clear again in Rule 64B16-27.103, which states that only a pharmacist or registered pharmacy intern acting under the supervision of a pharmacist may accept an oral prescription of any nature.
   b. interpreting a prescription or medication order for therapeutic acceptability and appropriateness;
   c. conducting the final verification of dosage and directions;
   d. engaging in prospective drug review;
   e. monitoring prescription usage;
   f. overriding clinical alerts;
   g. transferring a prescription;
   h. preparing a copy of a prescription or reading a prescription to any person for purposes of providing reference concerning treatment of the person or animal for whom the prescription is written;
      Note: Similar language is also found in Rule 64B16-27.103.
   i. engaging in patient counseling;
   j. receiving therapy or blood product procedures in a permitted nuclear pharmacy;
   k. engaging in any other act that requires the exercise of a pharmacist's professional judgment.

STUDY TIP: These are two separate rules that both try to describe functions or tasks that only a pharmacist may perform. While they are not identical, they do not appear to conflict. Regardless, it is important to know what duties or functions may only be performed by a pharmacist.

B. **Pharmacy Technicians**
   1. **Delegable and Non-Delegable Tasks (Rule 64B16-27.420)**
      This rule sets forth those tasks that a pharmacist may delegate to a pharmacy technician. These include:
      a. Data entry;
      b. Labeling of preparations and prescriptions;

c. Retrieval of prescription files, patient files and profiles, and other similar records pertaining to the practice of pharmacy;
  d. Counting, weighing, measuring, and pouring of prescription medication or stock legend drugs and controlled substances, including the filling of automated medication systems;
  e. Initiating communication to confirm a patient's name, medication, strength, quantity, directions, number of refills, and date of last fill;
  f. Initiating communication with a prescribing practitioner or their agent to obtain clarification on missing or illegible dates, prescriber name, brand or generic preference, quantity, license numbers, or DEA registration numbers;

STUDY TIP: A pharmacy technician may initiate the communication with the prescriber to clarify or confirm the things listed in e. and f., but only a pharmacist (or intern) may receive a new verbal prescription or interpret a prescription or medication order for therapeutic acceptability and appropriateness. If, in the process of clarifying, there is a change in the medication strength, or directions for use, the technician would need to let the pharmacist accept those changes as a verbal order.

  g. Accepting an authorization to refill an existing prescription that has no refills;
  h. Receiving of diagnostic orders only in a nuclear pharmacy;
  i. Organizing or participating in a continuous quality improvement meeting or program;
  j. Participating in a monitoring program to remove deteriorated pharmaceuticals to a quarantine area;
  Note: This appears to be applicable to nuclear pharmacies, or it may include expired drugs in a pharmacy.
  k. Performing any other mechanical, technical, or administrative tasks which do not constitute the practice of pharmacy.
2. Delegation to and Supervision of Pharmacy Technicians (Rule 64B16-27.4001)
  a. Delegation: A pharmacist shall not delegate more tasks than he or she can personally supervise and ensure

compliance with this rule. A pharmacist may delegate those nondiscretionary delegable tasks in Rule 64B16-27.420 above to registered pharmacy technicians (registered with the Board) or pharmacy technicians in training (technicians who are receiving practical training in board-approved pharmacy technician training programs who are not required to be registered with the Board).

    b. Supervision: Delegated tasks must be performed under the direct supervision of a pharmacist who shall make certain all applicable state and federal laws, including but not limited to confidentiality, are fully observed. The supervising pharmacist, in consultation with the prescription department manager or consultant pharmacist of record, will determine the appropriate methods of supervision based on the following definitions and requirements. No other person, permittee, or licensee shall interfere with the exercise of the supervising pharmacist's independent professional judgment in determining the supervision of delegated tasks.

    c. "Direct supervision" means supervision by a pharmacist who is readily and immediately available at all times the delegated tasks are being performed.

    d. "Readily and immediately available" means the pharmacist and pharmacy technician(s) are on the same physical premises, or if not, technology is used to enable real-time, two-way communications between the pharmacist and technician.

    e. Use of Technology
        (1) A pharmacist may employ technological means to communicate with or observe pharmacy technicians.
        (2) A pharmacist shall make certain all applicable state and federal laws, including but not limited to confidentiality, are fully observed when utilizing technological means of communication and observation.

STUDY TIP: These provisions authorize remote supervision of pharmacy technicians, including technicians working at home or other locations.

  3. Pharmacy Technician Ratio (Rule 64B16-27.410)
    a. General Rule—A pharmacist shall not supervise more than one registered pharmacy technician; nor shall a

pharmacy allow a supervision ratio of more than one registered pharmacy technician to one pharmacist unless specifically authorized to do so under this rule.

STUDY TIP: This language is inexplicably still in the rule, so it is included in this book, but the rule later specifically authorizes a 3:1, 6:1, or 8:1 ratio. So despite this language, it is incorrect to state that the ratio of registered pharmacy technicians to pharmacists is 1:1. See below.

    b. Six to One (6:1) Ratio—Any pharmacy or pharmacist may allow a supervision ratio of up to 6 registered pharmacy technicians to one pharmacist as long as the pharmacist or registered pharmacy technicians are not engaged in sterile compounding.

    c. Three to One (3:1) Ratio—Any pharmacy or pharmacist engaged in sterile compounding shall not exceed a ratio of 3 registered pharmacy technicians to one pharmacist.

STUDY TIP: This ratio only applies to pharmacists and technicians engaged in sterile compounding and does not affect the technician ratios for other activities not involving sterile compounding in areas of the pharmacy separated from the sterile compounding area. In other words, a pharmacy could have 3 technicians involved in sterile compounding supervised by a single pharmacist and 6 additional technicians in a separate area involved in other dispensing being supervised by another pharmacist.

    d. Eight-to-One (8:1) Ratio—A pharmacy may allow a supervision ratio of 8 registered pharmacy technicians to 1 pharmacist if the pharmacy is a non-dispensing pharmacy or, if it is a dispensing pharmacy, it may utilize an 8:1 ratio in any area physically separate (by a permanent wall or barrier) from the area where drugs are dispensed and there is no sterile compounding taking place.

STUDY TIP: This would apply to a call center pharmacy or remote order processing pharmacy that does not dispense medication.

C. Pharmacy Interns
    1. No intern shall perform any acts relating to the filling, compounding, or dispensing of medicinal drugs unless done

under the direct and immediate supervision of a Florida licensed pharmacist.
2. This implies that a registered pharmacy intern can perform the same acts as a pharmacist (except making the final check of a prescription) when under the direct and immediate supervision of a Florida licensed pharmacist. This would include those duties that a pharmacy technician cannot perform, such as counseling patients, receiving verbal prescriptions, etc.

STUDY TIP: There is no maximum ratio of interns to pharmacists except when an intern is performing immunizations and for foreign pharmacy graduate interns when a 1:1 ratio applies.

II. **Laws and Rules for All Pharmacy Permits or Applicable to Pharmacists in Any Location**
Note: These provisions appear to apply regardless of the practice location of the pharmacist because, unless otherwise noted, they do not reference a particular type of pharmacy permit, such as a community pharmacy or institutional pharmacy. For that reason, these sections are listed here rather than under a specific type of permit, even though it is likely that some of these practices only take place in specific types of practice settings, and some of these rules seem to be clearly written only for community pharmacies.
   A. Administration of Vaccines and Epinephrine Auto-injection (§ 465.189)
      1. A certified pharmacist (or certified registered intern) may administer vaccines to adults under a written protocol with a supervising physician.
      Note: Unlike some other states, the protocol is between the supervising physician and a pharmacist, not a pharmacy.
      2. To obtain certification, a pharmacist (or registered intern) must complete at least 20 hours of continuing education concerning the safe and effective administration of vaccines, including cardiopulmonary resuscitation (CPR) training. *See Rules 64B16-26.1031 and 64B16-26.1032 for details on certification application and training program*
      3. To maintain immunization certification, a pharmacist must complete 3 hours of continuing education during each two-year renewal period. *See § 465.009(6)*

4. Immunizations or vaccines authorized:
   a. Immunizations or vaccines listed in the Adult Immunization Schedule by the U.S. Centers for Disease Control and Prevention as of February 1, 2015. This includes:
      (1) Influenza
      (2) Tetanus, Diphtheria, Pertussis (Td/Tdap)
      (3) Human papillomavirus (HPV)
      (4) Zoster
      (5) Measles, mumps, rubella (MMR)
      (6) Pneumococcal 13-valent conjugate (PCV13)
      (7) Pneumococcal polysaccharide (PPSV23)
      (8) Meningococcal
      (9) Hepatitis A
      (10) Hepatitis B
      (11) Haemophilus influenzae type b (Hib)
      Note: Vaccines added to the recommended schedule by the CDC after February 1, 2015, can only be authorized by the Board if they issue a new rule. In 2016, Meningococcal B (MenB) was added. In 2018, Zoster Vaccine Recombinant, Adjuvanted was added. See Rule 64B16-27.630
   b. Immunizations or vaccines recommended by the U.S. Centers for Disease Control and Prevention for international travel as of July 1, 2015.
      Note: Yellow fever vaccinations require additional qualification to administer the immunization and issuance of a stamp by the Florida Bureau of Epidemiology.
   c. Immunizations or vaccines approved by the Board in response to a state of emergency declared by the Governor.
5. A pharmacist may not enter into a protocol unless he or she maintains at least $200,000 of professional liability insurance.
6. Immunization records must be maintained for 5 years.
7. A certified registered intern who administers a vaccine must be supervised by a certified pharmacist at a ratio of one pharmacist to one registered intern.

STUDY TIP: An intern does not need to enter into a protocol with a physician to provide immunizations, but must be certified to provide immunizations and be under the supervision of a pharmacist who is also certified to administer immunizations.

8. Florida has a statewide immunization registry, the State Health Online Tracking System (SHOTS). It is a centralized online immunization registry that helps parents, healthcare providers, and schools keep track of immunization records for children. According to the Florida Department of Health's website, Florida pharmacists are required to report all vaccinations to the SHOTS program even though they can only provide immunizations to adults. *See https://flshots users.com/pharmacists*

STUDY TIP: Florida allows certified pharmacists and interns to administer any CDC-recommended vaccine but only to patients 18 years of age or older. Florida is one of only a few states that restrict pharmacists from administering vaccines to children.

Note: HHS has authorized all pharmacists to provide immunizations to children ages 3–18 if certain conditions are met during the COVID-19 pandemic; however, it is not likely that the MPJE will include questions on temporary rules related to the COVID-19 pandemic.

B. Standards of Practice—Continuous Quality Improvement (CQI) Program (Rule 64B16-27.300)
   1. "Continuous Quality Improvement Program" means a system of standards and procedures to identify and evaluate quality-related events and improve patient care.
   2. "Quality Related Event" means the inappropriate dispensing or administration of a prescribed medication, including:
      a. a variation from the prescriber's prescription order, including but not limited to:
         (1) incorrect drug;
         (2) incorrect drug strength;
         (3) incorrect dosage form;
         (4) incorrect patient; or
         (5) inadequate or incorrect packaging, labeling, or directions; or
      b. a failure to identify and manage:
         (1) overutilization or underutilization;
         (2) therapeutic duplication;
         (3) drug-disease contraindications;
         (4) drug-drug interactions;
         (5) incorrect drug dosage or duration of treatment;
         (6) drug allergy interactions; or
         (7) clinical abuse/misuse.

3. Each pharmacy shall establish a CQI program, which shall be described in the pharmacy's policy and procedure manual and must contain:
   a. A CQI Committee that reviews quality-related events at least every three months;
   b. A planned process to record, measure, assess, and improve the quality of patient care; and
   c. A procedure reviewing quality-related events.
4. At a minimum, the review shall consider the effects on quality of the pharmacy system due to staffing levels, workflow, and technological support.
5. As part of the CQI program, each pharmacy shall assure that all reasonable steps have been taken to remedy any problem for the patient.
6. Each quality-related event shall be documented.
7. Records maintained as a component of a pharmacy CQI program are confidential under § 766.101 Florida Statutes (Medical Review Committees—immunity from liability). Records are considered peer review documents and are not subject to discovery in civil litigation or administrative actions.

STUDY TIP: The prescription department manager or consultant pharmacist of record is responsible for ensuring that a pharmacy has an operating CQI program and that all CQI activities are documented.

C. Pharmacy Technician Policies and Training (Rule 64B16-27.410(2) and (3))
   1. All pharmacies must establish and maintain a policy and procedure manual regarding the number of registered pharmacy technician positions that includes the specific scope of delegable tasks of the technicians, job descriptions, and task protocols. The manual must include the following topics:
      a. Supervision by a pharmacist;
      b. Minimum qualifications of registered pharmacy technicians;
      c. In-service education or ongoing training and demonstration of competency;
      d. General duties and responsibilities;
      e. All functions related to prescription processing;
      f. All functions related to prescription drug and controlled substance ordering and inventory control, documentation, and recordkeeping;

- g. All functions related to retrieval of prescription files, patient files, patient profile information, and other records;
- h. All delegable tasks and non-delegable tasks per 64B16-27.420 (*See Pharmacy Technician section above*);
- i. Confidentiality and privacy laws and rules;
- j. Prescription refill and renewal authorizations;
- k. Functions related to automated pharmacy systems; and
- l. Continuous Quality Improvement program.
2. Pharmacies must maintain documentation that is signed by the registered pharmacy technician, acknowledging the technician has reviewed the policy and procedure manual within 90 days from the date hired.
3. Pharmacies must maintain documentation that demonstrates registered pharmacy technicians have received training in their established job description, delegable tasks, task protocols, and policies and procedures in the specific pharmacy. This documentation must be one of the following:
   - a. Certification by the supervising licensee (i.e., pharmacist);
   - b. Certification by an instructor, trainer, or other similar person;
   - c. Training attendance logs or completion certificates accompanied by an outline of the material addresses; or
   - d. Exam or written questionnaires.

D. Prescription Area Accessible for Inspection (Rule 64B16-28.101)
1. The prescription department, compounding room, or any other place where prescriptions are compounded, filled, processed, accepted, dispensed, or stored in each pharmacy shall be so situated and located to allow authorized agents and employees of the Department or other persons authorized by law to enter and inspect the pharmacy.
2. A pharmacy shall be inspected twice during the first year of operation.
3. A pharmacy which has had passing inspections for the most current three years and no discipline during that time shall be inspected every two years.
4. A pharmacy which fails to pass an inspection, or which is disciplined during the two-year inspection cycle, will be inspected annually until it achieves passing inspections and no discipline for the most current three-year period.

5. Authorized agents of the Department or other persons authorized by law may inspect invoices, shipping tickets, or any other document pertaining to the transfer of drugs from or to all pharmacies.

E. Sink and Running Water; Sufficient Space; Refrigeration; Sanitation; Equipment; and Library Requirements (Rule 64B16-28.102)
   1. The prescription department of each pharmacy must have:
      a. a sink in workable condition and running water accessible to the prescription counter;
      b. sufficient shelf, drawer, or cabinet space for the neat and orderly storage of pharmaceutical stock, prescription containers, prescription labels, and all required equipment;
      c. sufficient walking space and work counter space to allow employees to adequately, safely, and accurately fulfill their duties;
      d. adequate sanitation to ensure the prescription department is operating under clean, sanitary, uncrowded, and healthy conditions; and
      e. other equipment as is necessary to meet the needs of the professional practice of the pharmacy.
   2. The prescription department of each pharmacy must have the following items:
      a. A current pharmacy reference compendium such as the United States Pharmacopeia/National Formulary, the U.S. Dispensatory, United States Pharmacopeia Drug Information (USP DI), Remington's Science and Practice of Pharmacy, Facts and Comparisons, or equivalent.
      b. A current copy of the laws and rules governing the practice of pharmacy.
      c. These library requirements may be maintained in a readily available electronic format.

STUDY TIP: Knowing the library requirements in a pharmacy is a listed MPJE Competency. These listed references are examples. The "or equivalent" language would allow a pharmacy to have other references, and online access to these references meets the requirement.

F. All Permits—Labels and Labeling of Medicinal Drugs (Rule 28.108)
   Note: Although this rule is labeled "all permits," specific sections of the rule are applicable only to specific types of pharmacy permits.

Those label requirements have been omitted from this section and moved to the rules for the specific type of pharmacy permit.

1. Label Requirements for Drugs Dispensed to a Patient
   a. Name and address of the pharmacy
      Note: Telephone number of the pharmacy is not listed in the rule.
   b. Date of dispensing
   c. Serial number (prescription number)
   d. Name of the patient or, if the patient is an animal, the name of the owner and species of animal
   e. Name of the prescriber
   f. Name of the drug dispensed
      Note: Strength and quantity is not listed in the rule.
   g. Directions for use
   h. An expiration date or beyond-use date. The expiration date must be the date provided by the manufacturer. The beyond-use date may not exceed the expiration date and cannot be greater than one year from the date dispensed. "Discard-after date" or "Do Not Use-after date" are considered beyond-use dates. *See also § 465.0255*

STUDY TIP: Note that the expiration date is defined as the date from the manufacturer while the beyond-use date cannot be more than one year. Although the rules allow a pharmacy to put either on the label, most pharmacies use a beyond-use date unless the product is being dispensed in the manufacturer's original packaging.

   i. If the drug is a controlled substance, the federal transfer warning is also required. *See Chapter 2*

STUDY TIP: The required elements on a prescription label are a good example of the type of information that is done automatically by pharmacy computer systems, but for the MPJE it is helpful to memorize the specific requirements.

2. Label Requirements for Customized Medication Packages
   Note: Customized Medication Packages are packages prepared by a pharmacist for a specific patient that is a series of containers containing two or more solid oral dosage forms. They are used to improve patient compliance by packaging together two or more drugs that will be taken at the same time. They may be used with consent of the patient or patient's agent.

      a. Name, address, and telephone number of the pharmacy
      b. Date of preparation of the customized medication package
      c. Serial number (prescription number) of the customized medication package and a separate serial number (prescription number) for each drug dispensed
      d. Patient's name
      e. Name of each prescriber
      f. Directions for use and any cautionary statements required for each drug
      g. Storage instructions
      h. Name, strength, quantity, and physical description of each drug product
      i. A beyond-use date that is not more than 60 days from the date of the preparation of the customized medication package. If any of the drugs in the customized medication package have an expiration date that is less than 60 days from the date prepared, that date shall be the beyond-use date for the customized medication package.

STUDY TIP: Be sure to know the differences in the labeling requirements between regular prescriptions and customized medication packages. The telephone number of the pharmacy and strength and quantity of the drug seem to be more of an oversight by the Board when drafting the rule, but the beyond-use date and the requirement for a physical description of the product are differences that are clearly intentional. Also, note that if these customized medication packages are used in nursing homes, the patient-specific information does not have to appear on each individual label. *See Labeling of Drugs for Inpatient of a Nursing Home rule later in this chapter*

  G. Record Maintenance System for All Pharmacy Permits (Rule 64B16-28.140)
     1. All original prescriptions shall be retained for a period of not less than 4 years from the date of last filling.

STUDY TIP: This is longer than the two-year requirement for controlled substance prescriptions required by DEA. Also note that it is four years from the date of last filling, not four years from the date the prescription was issued or first filled.

2. Pharmacies may use an electronic imaging recordkeeping system instead of keeping original prescriptions as long as the system is capable of capturing, storing, and reproducing an exact image of the prescription, including the reverse side if necessary. Such images must be retained for 4 years from the date of last filling.

   Note: Although Florida law allows this for all prescriptions, DEA still requires original written controlled substance prescriptions to be maintained using the two or three file system described in Chapter 2.

3. Details regarding records maintained in a data processing (computer) system include:
   a. Information stored in a computer system must be backed up at least weekly.
   b. Computer systems must be able to produce an audit trail of drug usage for the preceding 4 years.
   c. Records of dispensing—Computer systems must have the capability of producing a daily hard-copy printout of all prescriptions filled or refilled containing the following information:
      (1) Prescription number;
      (2) Date of dispensing;
      (3) Patient name;
      (4) Prescribing practitioner's name;
      (5) Name and strength of product dispensed (manufacturer if generic);
      (6) Quantity dispensed;
      (7) Initials or identification of dispensing pharmacist; and
      (8) If not immediately retrievable via CRT display (i.e., the monitor or computer screen), must also include patient's address, prescriber's address, prescriber's DEA number if for controlled substance, quantity prescribed if different from quantity dispensed, date of issuance of prescription if different from date of dispensing, and total number of refills dispensed to date.

      Note: Bonus points if you know what a CRT display is. This rule was written when computers only had Cathode Ray Tube (CRT) monitors. These are no longer made.

- **d.** If a pharmacy chooses to print the daily hard copy, the following requirements must be met:
    - **(1)** It must be produced (printed) within 72 hours of date drugs were dispensed.
    - **(2)** Each individual pharmacist who dispenses or refills a prescription shall verify that the data is correct by dating and signing (no initials) the daily hard copy within 7 days.
- **e.** Instead of printing the daily hard copy, a pharmacy may maintain a logbook in which each individual pharmacist signs a statement each day attesting that the information entered into the computer is correct.
  Note: This is what most pharmacies do. They do not usually print out a complete daily hard copy.
- **f.** The computer system must be able to print a hard copy on demand by an authorized agent of the Department of Health. If no printer is on site, the hard-copy printout must be provided within 48 hours or it is considered a failure to keep and maintain records.

STUDY TIP: The computer system recordkeeping rules are taken from DEA rules, but Florida rules apply them to all prescription records maintained in the computer system, not just controlled substances. Also note, if a pharmacy is not printing a daily hard copy (and most pharmacies are not), the computer must be able to produce records on demand or within 48 hours. This is slightly different than the requirement to print a "summary record" of controlled substances dispensed in the past 60 days by prescriber or patient in Rule 64B16-27.831, which must be produced within 72 hours.

- **H.** Centralized Prescription Filling (§ 465.0265 and Rule 64B16-28.450)
    1. A pharmacy may perform centralized prescription filling for another pharmacy if they have the same owner or have a contract with the other pharmacy.
    2. Each pharmacy (the originating pharmacy and the central fill pharmacy) must have a policy and procedure manual that includes the following information:
        - **a.** A description of how each pharmacy will comply with federal and state laws, rules, and regulations.
        - **b.** The procedure for maintaining appropriate records to identify the pharmacist responsible for dispensing the prescription and counseling the patient.

    c. Procedures for tracking the prescription during each stage of filling and dispensing.
    d. The procedure for identifying on the prescription label all pharmacies involved in filling and dispensing the prescription.
    e. Policies and procedures for providing adequate security to protect the confidentiality and integrity of patient information.
    f. The procedure for implementing and operating a quality assurance program.
    g. The types of medication that may and may not be filled by the central fill pharmacy.
    h. The procedures for securely transporting the filled prescriptions from the central fill pharmacy to the originating pharmacy.
    i. The specific services provided and the duties and responsibilities of each pharmacy.
3. Labeling
    a. Both the central fill pharmacy and the originating pharmacy shall be identified on the label.
    b. The originating pharmacy must be identified on the label by name and address.
    c. The central fill pharmacy may be identified on the label by a code.
4. See Rule 64B16-28.450 for details on transmission of information between the originating pharmacy and the central fill pharmacy.
5. Delivering prescriptions from a central fill pharmacy directly to a patient.
    a. A community central fill pharmacy may deliver non-controlled medications for an originating pharmacy directly to a patient if the pharmacies have a pharmacist available 40 hours a week, either in person or via two-way communication technology (telephone, etc.), and a toll-free number to provide counseling.
    b. A central fill pharmacy may not deliver controlled substances directly to a patient.

STUDY TIP: This is an important distinction. DEA only allows central fill pharmacies to send filled prescriptions to the originating pharmacy.

       c. When a central fill pharmacy delivers a filled prescription directly to a patient, it is not considered dispensing.
Note: This is because it is treated more like the central fill pharmacy is delivering the prescription on behalf of the originating pharmacy.
       d. A Class II Institutional central fill pharmacy may only deliver medication to the originating pharmacy.
   6. A community pharmacy which acts only as a central fill pharmacy and notifies the Board is exempt from requirements for a patient counseling area (Rule 64B16-28.1035), signage requirements (Rule 64B16-28.109(1)), and operating hours (Rule 64B16-28.1081).

I. Other Rules Applicable to All Pharmacy Permits
   1. Transfer of Medicinal Drugs; Change of Ownership (Rule 64B16-28.203)
       a. Must provide transfer information to the Board of Pharmacy.
       b. Must complete an inventory of all controlled substances.
       c. Transfers of Schedule II drugs must be done with a DEA 222 form.
   2. Outdated pharmaceuticals (Rule 64B16-28.110)
All outdated, damaged, deteriorated, misbranded, or adulterated prescription drugs shall be removed or quarantined from active stock.
   3. Promoting sale of certain drugs prohibited (§ 465.024)
No pharmacist, owner, or employee of a retail drug establishment shall use any communication media to promote or advertise the use or sale of any controlled substance appearing in any schedule in Chapter 893.
Note: This says "employees of a retail drug establishment" but it appears to apply to all pharmacists regardless of practice location, so it is included under requirements for all pharmacy permits.
   4. Information Disclosure (§ 465.0244)
Every pharmacy shall make available in its website a hyperlink to the health information that is disseminated by the Agency for Health Care Administration, which provides a consumer-friendly, internet-based platform that allows a consumer to research the cost of healthcare services and procedures and allows for price comparison. This website can be found at *https://pricing.floridahealthfinder.gov*

5. Permits; Single Entity; Single Location (Rule 64B16-28.113)
   a. Only a single entity may obtain a pharmacy permit at a single location.
   b. A single location is defined as a contiguous area under the control of the permit holder but cannot include an area more than ½ mile from the central location.
   c. A public thoroughfare (i.e., street, public walkway, etc.) does not break the area contiguity.
   Note: This is to allow a campus DEA registration. Pharmacists should be certain that the area covered by a permit is clear and that the pharmacy permit and DEA registration are consistent.
6. Rebates Prohibited (§ 465.185 and Rules 64B16-27.1042 and 64B16-27.104(3))
   a. It is unlawful for any person to pay or receive any commission, bonus, kickback, or rebate or engage in any split-fee arrangement in any form whatsoever with any physician, surgeon, organization, agency, or person, either directly or indirectly, for patients referred to a pharmacy.
   b. Rule 64B16-27.1042 provides detailed examples of prohibited acts, such as providing supplies or equipment, including computers, fax machines, etc., to a facility.
   c. No pharmacist, pharmacy, employee, or agent thereof shall enter into or engage in any agreement or arrangement with any physician, other practitioner, nursing home, or extended care facility for the payment or acceptance of compensation in any form or type for the recommending of the professional services of either; or enter into a rebate or percentage rental agreement of any kind, whereby in any way a patient's free choice of a pharmacist or pharmacy is or may be limited.
7. Human Trafficking Sign (Florida Statute § 546.0341)
   a. Legislation passed in 2019 requires pharmacists to post in their place of work (i.e., in the pharmacy), in a conspicuous place accessible to employees, a sign at least 11 in. by 15 in. size, printed in a clearly legible font and in at least a 32-point type, which substantially states in English and Spanish:
   "If you or someone you know is being forced to engage in an activity and cannot leave, whether it is prostitution,

housework, farm work, factory work, retail work, restaurant work, or any other activity, call the National Human Trafficking Resource Center at 888-373-7888 or text INFO or HELP to 233-733 to access help and services. Victims of slavery and human trafficking are protected under United States and Florida law."
  b. This must be completed by January 1, 2021.

III. **Pharmacists Order For Medicinal Drugs, Drug Therapy Management, Collaborative Practice, & Test and Treat**
  A. Pharmacist's Order for Medicinal Drugs (§ 465.186) *Note: This law was an early attempt passed in the 1980s to provide limited pharmacist prescriptive authority. The law is not used in practice very often anymore, but it is still an active law, and you could be asked questions about it on the MPJE.*
   1. The Florida Pharmacy Act provides for a committee to develop a formulary of medicinal drugs that a pharmacist may order (i.e., prescribe) and dispense as well as a dispensing procedure. Drugs must fall under one of the following categories:
   a. Any medicinal drug of single or multiple ingredients in any strength whose active ingredient(s) have been approved for OTC sale.
   b. Any medicinal drug recommended by an FDA Advisory Panel for transfer to OTC status pending approval by FDA.
   c. Any medicinal drug containing an antihistamine or decongestant as a single active ingredient or in combination.
   d. Any medicinal drug containing fluoride in any strength.
   e. Any medicinal drug containing lindane in any strength.
   f. Any OTC proprietary drug approved for reimbursement by the Florida Medicaid program.
   g. Any topical anti-infectives excluding eye and ear anti-infectives.
   2. Drugs on formulary may only be dispensed by the pharmacist ordering the drug and shall not be refilled, nor shall another drug be ordered for the same condition unless consistent with the dispensing procedures.

3. Drugs provided must be labeled with the following information:
   a. Name of the pharmacist ordering the medication;
   b. Name and address of the pharmacy dispensing the drug;
   c. Date of dispensing;
   d. Prescription number;
   e. Name of the patient;
   f. Directions for use;
   g. Clear statement that order cannot be refilled;
   h. Trade name or generic name [from Rule 64B16-27.210(6)]; and
   i. Quantity dispensed [from Rule 64B16-27.210(6)].
4. Any pharmacist providing these services shall be eligible for reimbursement by third-party plans when so provided by contract.
5. General terms and conditions to be followed by a pharmacist when ordering and dispensing approved medicinal drugs (Rule 64B16-27.210):
   a. May not order injectable drugs.
   b. May not order drugs for pregnant patients or nursing mothers.
   c. Quantity cannot exceed a 34-day supply or standard course of treatment.
   d. Patients shall be advised that they should seek the advice of an appropriate healthcare provider if their present condition, symptom, or complaint does not improve upon completion of the drug regimen.
   e. Directions for use shall not exceed the manufacturer's recommended dosage.
   f. May only perform service in a Florida permitted pharmacy.
   g. The pharmacist must create a prescription.
   h. The pharmacist must maintain a patient profile, separate from the prescription order, and shall date and initial all profile entries.
      (1) Such profiles shall be maintained for 4 years.
      (2) Required information to be in patient profile includes medical history, current complaint, drug ordered, etc.
6. Formulary of Medicinal Drugs Which May Be Ordered by Pharmacists Rule (64B16-27.220)

FORMULARY OF MEDICINAL DRUGS WHICH MAY BE ORDERED BY PHARMACISTS

Oral analgesics for mild to moderate pain and menstrual cramps for patients with no history of peptic ulcer disease (limited to a six-day supply)
- Magnesium salicylate/phenyltoloxamine citrate
- Acetylsalicylic acid (zero order release, long-acting tablets)
- Choline salicylate and magnesium salicylate
- Naproxen sodium
- Naproxen
- Ibuprofen

Urinary analgesics
- Phenazopyridine, not exceeding a two-day supply

Otic analgesics
- Antipyrene 5.4%, benzocaine 1.4%, glycerin

Anti-nausea preparations:
- Meclizine up to 25 mg, except for patients taking a CNS depressant
- Scopolamine not exceeding 1.5 mg per dermal patch

Antihistamines—for patients 6 years of age or older
- Diphenhydramine
- Carbinoxamine
- Pyriliamine
- Dexchlorpheniramine
- Brompheniramine

Decongestants for patients 6 years of age or older
- Phenylephrine
- Azatadine

Topical antifungals/antibacterials
- Iodochlorhydroxyquin with 0.5% hydrocortisone (not exceeding 20 g)
- Haloprogin 1%
- Clotrimazole topical cream and lotion
- Erythromycin topical

Topical anti-inflammatory preparations
- Hydrocortisone not exceeding 2.5%

Otic antifungal/antibacterial
- Acetic acid 2% in aluminum acetate solution

Keratolytics
    Salicylic acid 16.7% and lactic acid 16.7% to be applied to warts except for patients under 2 and those with diabetes or impaired circulation
    Vitamins with fluoride (not including vitamins with folic acid exceeding 0.9 mg)
    Medicinal drug shampoos containing lindane—not more than 4 oz.
Ophthalmics
    Naphazoline 0.1%
Histamine H2 antagonists
    Cimetidine
    Famotidine
    Ranitidine
Topical antivirals
    Acyclovir ointment for treatment of herpes simplex of lips
    Penciclovir
Acne product
    Benzoyl peroxide

B. Drug Therapy Management (Rule 64B16-27.830) *Note: This rule was in place prior to when the newer Collaborative Practice and Test and Treat laws in C. and D. below were adopted.*

    1. This rule allows pharmacists to provide drug therapy management services in compliance with orders in a "Prescriber Care Plan" written by a physician, physician assistant, dentist, or podiatrist. *Note: APRNs are not included in this rule, but PAs are.*

    2. A "Prescriber Care Plan" is an individualized assessment of a patient and orders for specific drugs, laboratory tests, and other pharmaceutical services intended to be dispensed or executed by a pharmacist. It shall specify the conditions under which a pharmacist shall order laboratory tests, interpret laboratory values, execute drug therapy orders for a patient, and notify the prescriber.

    3. A pharmacist can provide Drug Therapy Management incidental to dispensing, as part of consulting on therapeutic values of drugs, or as part of managing and monitoring a patient's drug therapy.

4. Drug Therapy Management may only be provided under the auspices of a pharmacy permit that provides:
   a. A transferable patient care record, which includes a Prescriber Care Plan that includes a section noted as "orders" from a prescriber for each patient and progress notes;
   b. A pharmaceutical care area that is private, distinct, and partitioned from any area in which activities other than patient care activities occur and in which the pharmacist and patient can sit down; and
   c. A Continuous Quality Improvement program that includes standards and procedures to identify, evaluate, and constantly improve Drug Therapy Management Services.

C. Collaborative Practice (§ 465.1865 and Rules 64B16-31.001–64B16-31.007)
   1. This legislation, effective July 1, 2020, permits a certified pharmacist to enter into a collaborative practice agreement with a physician (D.O. or M.D.) for certain chronic health conditions.
   2. Chronic health condition means:
      a. Arthritis;
      b. Asthma;
      c. Chronic obstructive pulmonary diseases;
      d. Type 2 diabetes;
      e. Human immunodeficiency virus or acquired immune deficiency syndrome;
      f. Obesity; or
      g. Any other chronic condition adopted in rule by the board, in consultation with the Board of Medicine and Board of Osteopathic Medicine. In Rule 64B16-31.007, the Board adopted the following additional chronic conditions for which a pharmacist can provide services to patients under a Collaborative Pharmacy Practice Service Agreement:
         (1) Hyperlipidemia;
         (2) Hypertension;
         (3) Anti-coagulation management;
         (4) Nicotine dependence; and
         (5) Opioid use disorder.

3. To be certified, a pharmacist must, at a minimum:
   a. Hold an active and unencumbered license to practice pharmacy in this state.
   b. Have earned a degree of doctor of pharmacy or have completed 5 years of experience as a licensed pharmacist.
   c. Have completed an initial 20-hour course approved by the board, in consultation with the Board of Medicine and Board of Osteopathic Medicine, that includes, at a minimum, instruction on the following:
      (1) Performance of patient assessments;
      (2) Ordering, performing, and interpreting clinical and laboratory tests related to collaborative pharmacy practice;
      (3) Evaluating and managing diseases and health conditions in collaboration with other healthcare practitioners;
      (4) Any other area required by the board. In Rule 64B16-31.003, the Board adopted the following additional content areas and requirements for the initial certification course:
         i. Applicable laws and rules;
         ii. Writing and entering into a collaborative practice agreement;
         iii. No less than 8 hours of the course shall be offered through a live webinar or video conference;
         iv. A pharmacist who successfully completes a Board-approved collaborative practice certification course shall be awarded 20 hours of general continuing education credits; and
         v. The course may be provided by a provider who is accredited by the Accreditation Council for Pharmacy Education (ACPE), a program provider accredited to provide educational activities designated for the American Medical Association Physician's Recognition Award Category I credit, or a program provider approved by the American Osteopathic Association to offer continuing medical education credits.
   d. Maintain at least $250,000 of professional liability insurance coverage.

- e. File an application for Pharmacist Collaborative Practice Certification available on the Board's website.
- f. Have established a system to maintain records of all patients receiving services under a collaborative pharmacy practice agreement for a period of 5 years from each patient's most recent provision of service.
4. The terms and conditions of the collaborative pharmacy practice agreement must be appropriate to the pharmacist's training, and the services delegated to the pharmacist must be within the collaborating physician's scope of practice. A copy of the certification issued under this subsection must be included as an attachment to the collaborative pharmacy practice agreement.
    - a. A collaborative pharmacy practice agreement must include the following:
        - (1) Name of the collaborating physician's patient or patients for whom a pharmacist may provide services;
        - (2) Each chronic health condition to be collaboratively managed;
        - (3) Specific medicinal drug or drugs to be managed by the pharmacist for each patient;
        - (4) Circumstances under which the pharmacist may order or perform and evaluate laboratory or clinical tests;
        - (5) Conditions and events upon which the pharmacist must notify the collaborating physician and the manner and time frame in which such notification must occur;
        - (6) Beginning and ending dates for the collaborative pharmacy practice agreement and termination procedures, including procedures for patient notification and medical records transfers; and
        - (7) A statement that the collaborative pharmacy practice agreement may be terminated, in writing, by either party at any time.
    - b. A collaborative pharmacy practice agreement shall automatically terminate 2 years after execution if not renewed.
    - c. The pharmacist, along with the collaborating physician, must maintain on file the collaborative pharmacy

practice agreement at his or her practice location, and must make such agreements available to the department or board upon request or inspection.

    d. A pharmacist who enters into a collaborative pharmacy practice agreement must submit a copy of the signed agreement to the board before the agreement may be implemented.

5. Additional Requirements

    a. Prior to providing or implementing patient care services under a collaborative pharmacy practice agreement or immediately after the renewal of such an agreement, the pharmacist shall submit the executed agreement to the Board's office through the pharmacist's online licensure account.

    b. In the event of an addendum to the material terms of an existing collaborative practice agreement, the pharmacist shall maintain a copy of the addendum and the initial agreement.

    Note: Material items include required elements in 4.a. above.

6. A pharmacist may not:

    a. Modify or discontinue medicinal drugs prescribed by a healthcare practitioner with whom he or she does not have a collaborative pharmacy practice agreement.

    b. Enter into a collaborative pharmacy practice agreement while acting as an employee without the written approval of the owner of the pharmacy.

7. A physician may not delegate the authority to initiate or prescribe a controlled substance as described to a pharmacist.

8. A pharmacist who practices under a collaborative pharmacy practice agreement must complete an 8-hour continuing education course approved by the board that addresses issues related to collaborative pharmacy practice each biennial licensure renewal, in addition to the general continuing education requirements. A pharmacist must submit confirmation of having completed such course when applying for licensure renewal. A pharmacist who fails to comply with this subsection shall be prohibited from practicing under a collaborative pharmacy practice agreement under this section.

9. A pharmacist practicing under a collaborative pharmacy practice agreement who diagnoses or suspects the existence of a disease of public health significance shall immediately report the fact to the Department of Health.

Note: See the Florida Department of Health website for a list of reportable diseases/conditions.

D. Testing or screening for and treatment of minor, nonchronic health conditions (§ 465.1895 and Board Rules 64B16-31.033–64B16-31.043)
   1. This legislation, effective July 1, 2020, allows a certified pharmacist to test or screen for and treat minor, nonchronic health conditions within the framework of an established written protocol with a supervising physician (D.O. or M.D.).
   2. A minor, nonchronic health condition is typically a short-term condition that is generally managed with minimal treatment or self-care, and includes:
      a. Influenza;
      b. Streptococcus;
      c. Lice;
      d. Skin conditions, such as ringworm and athlete's foot; and
      e. Minor, uncomplicated infections.
   3. To test and treat under this section, a pharmacist must:
      a. Hold an active and unencumbered license to practice pharmacy in the state.
      b. Hold a certification issued by the board to test and screen for and treat minor, nonchronic health conditions, in accordance with requirements established by the board in rule in consultation with the Board of Medicine and Board of Osteopathic Medicine. An application for Pharmacist Test and Treat Certification is available on the Board's website.
         (1) The certification must require a pharmacist to complete, on a onetime basis, a 20-hour education course approved by the board in consultation with the Board of Medicine and the Board of Osteopathic Medicine.
         (2) The course, at a minimum, must address patient assessments; point-of-care testing procedures; safe and effective treatment of minor, nonchronic health conditions; and identification of contraindications.

In Rule 64B16-31.035, the Board adopted the following additional requirements for the course content:
  i. Applicable laws and rules;
  ii. Writing and entering into a written protocol;
  iii. No less than 8 hours of the course shall be offered through a live webinar or video conference;
  iv. A pharmacist who successfully completes a Board-approved test-and-treat certification course shall be awarded 20 hours of general continuing education credits; and
  v. The course may be provided by a provider who is accredited by the Accreditation Council for Pharmacy Education (ACPE, a program provider accredited to provide educational activities designated for the American Medical Association Physician's Recognition Award Category I credit, or a program provider approved by the American Osteopathic Association to offer continuing medical education credits.
  c. Maintain at least $250,000 of liability coverage.
4. The Board shall adopt, by rule, a formulary of medicinal drugs that a pharmacist may prescribe for the minor, non-chronic health conditions.
  a. The formulary must include medicinal drugs approved by the United States Food and Drug Administration which are indicated for treatment of the minor, non-chronic health condition. The formulary may not include any controlled substances.
  b. Per Board Rule 64B16-31.039, the formulary of drugs a pharmacist may prescribe pursuant to a written test and treat protocol includes all medicinal drugs approved by the FDA and all compounded medicinal drugs that utilize only active pharmaceutical ingredients approved by the FDA.

STUDY TIP: Medicinal drugs are prescription drugs, but not controlled substances.

---

5. A pharmacist who tests or screens for and treats minor, non-chronic health conditions may use any tests that may guide

diagnosis or clinical decision making in which the Centers for Medicare and Medicaid Services have determined qualifies for a waiver under the federal Clinical Laboratory Improvement Amendments of 1988, or the federal rules adopted thereunder, or any established screening procedures that can safely be performed by a pharmacist.
6. A pharmacist testing or screening for and treating minor, nonchronic health conditions under a written protocol who diagnoses or suspects the existence of a disease of public health significance shall immediately report the fact to the Department of Health.
Note: See the Florida Department of Health website for a list of reportable diseases/conditions.
7. The written protocol must include, at a minimum, the following information:
   a. Specific categories of patients who the pharmacist is authorized to test or screen for and treat minor, nonchronic health conditions;
   b. The physician's instructions for obtaining relevant patient medical history for the purpose of identifying disqualifying health conditions, adverse reactions, and contraindications to the approved course of treatment;
   c. The physician's instructions for the treatment of minor, nonchronic health conditions based on the patient's age, symptoms, and test results, including negative results;
   d. A process and schedule for the physician to review the pharmacist's actions under the protocol; and
   e. A process and schedule for the pharmacist to notify the physician of the patient's condition, tests administered, test results, and course of treatment.
8. Additional requirements:
   a. Within 5 days of entering into a written protocol with a supervising physician, a pharmacist shall submit a copy of the written agreement to the Board of Pharmacy through the pharmacist's online licensure account.
   b. In the event an addendum is made to the material terms of an existing written protocol, the pharmacist shall maintain a copy of the addendum and the initial agreement.
   Note: Material items are those required elements of a protocol listed in 7. above.

      c. Upon request from a patient, a pharmacist shall furnish records to a healthcare practitioner designated by the patient within a reasonable time frame, not to exceed 5 days.

      d. A pharmacist must provide written information to a patient advising the patient to seek follow-up care with his or her primary care physician. This must be done:

          (1) Prior to performing testing, screening, or treatment services for the first time;

          (2) As outlined in the written protocol; and

          (3) When the pharmacist determines in his or her professional judgment that the patient should follow-up with his or her primary care provider.

      e. The pharmacy in which a pharmacist's tests and screens for and treats minor, nonchronic conditions must prominently display signage indicating that any patient receiving testing, screening, or treatment services is advised to seek follow-up care from his or her primary care physician.

IV. Community Pharmacies

Note: Many of the laws and rules in this section are worded to apply to all pharmacies, but they are most relevant to community pharmacies, so they are placed here for ease of learning. Provisions may be applicable to other practice sites such as hospital pharmacies that are dispensing to outpatients under a Limited Community Pharmacy Permit.

  A. Prescription Department Manager (Rules 64B16-27.104(5) and 64B16-27.450)

      1. All community pharmacies must have a licensed pharmacist who is designated as the Prescription Department Manager (PDM).

      2. The PDM is responsible for:

          a. maintaining all drug records;

          b. providing for the security of the prescription department; and

          c. ensuring the pharmacy's compliance with all statutes and rules.

      3. The Board shall not register a PDM as the manager of more than one pharmacy; however, the Board may grant an exception to this requirement upon application by the pharmacy and the PDM showing circumstances, such as proximity of

pharmacies and limited pharmacist workload, that would allow the manager to carry out all of the duties and responsibilities required of a PDM.
4. A community pharmacy shall continuously maintain a designated PDM at all times the pharmacy is open and operational.
5. Change of PDM
   a. No later than 10 days after a change in the designated PDM for a community pharmacy, both the pharmacy permittee and the newly designated PDM shall notify the Board of the change and the identity of the new PDM.
   b. A newly designated PDM must comply with the fingerprint requirements of § 465.0135 and 465.022.

B. Regulation of Daily Operating Hours; Commencement of Operations (Rule 64B16-28.1081)
1. A community pharmacy that commences to operate must have the prescription department open for a minimum of 20 hours per week.
2. A community pharmacy may delay the commencement of operations after receiving a permit by notifying the Board of Pharmacy, in writing, within 14 days of the election to delay commencement of operations and the reason for doing so.
3. A pharmacy that has delayed commencement of operations shall post a sign in block letters not less than 1 in. in height at the main entrance of the establishment stating that the pharmacy has not yet commenced operations and that medicinal drugs may not be sold nor prescriptions filled or dispensed.
4. Within 2 days of commencement of operations, the pharmacy shall notify the Board in writing that the pharmacy has commenced operations and the date of commencement.
5. Any pharmacy that fails to commence operations within 6 months of the date of receipt of the Florida pharmacy permit shall provide a written statement to the Board office, which shall include the reason(s) the pharmacy has not yet commenced operations, the efforts the pharmacy has made to commence operations, and the date the pharmacy expects to commence operations.
6. At the time a pharmacy commences operations, a sign in block letters not less than 1 in. in height stating the hours the prescription department is open each day shall be placed

at the main entrance of the establishment or at or near the place where prescriptions are dispensed.
7. Any pharmacy not open 40 hours per week must post the days and hours the pharmacy is open and information for after-hours access and shall also have a written policy and procedure for transferring a prescription or receiving an emergency dose pursuant to § 465.0275. *Note: § 465.0275 is the emergency refill law, so this probably should say "providing an emergency refill" rather than "receiving an emergency dose." Because of these requirements, it is difficult to have a community pharmacy that is open less than 40 hours per week unless a variance from this requirement is obtained.*

C. Prescription Department; Padlock; Closed (Rule 64B16-28.109)
1. A prescription department is considered closed whenever the establishment is open and a pharmacist is not present and on duty.
2. A sign with bold letters not less than 2 in. in height with the language "Prescription Department Closed" must be placed in the prescription department so that it may be easily read.
3. When the prescription department is closed, it shall be separated from the remainder of the establishment by a partition or other means of enclosure to prevent access and shall be securely locked. Only a pharmacist shall have the means to gain access to the prescription department, and no person other than a pharmacist may enter the department when it is closed.
4. A pharmacist may leave the prescription department for purposes of consulting or providing assistance to patients, attending to personal hygiene needs, taking a meal break, or providing other functions for which the pharmacist is responsible for.

D. Meal Break Rule (Rule 64B16-27.1001(6))
1. A pharmacist may take a meal break, not to exceed 30 minutes in length, during which time the prescription department is not considered closed.
2. A pharmacist is considered present and on duty during a meal break if the pharmacy posts a sign that indicates the specific hours of the day during which meal breaks may be taken by the pharmacist and assuring patients that a pharmacist is available on the premises for consultation upon

request during a meal break. *Note: This implies that a pharmacist may not leave the premises for a meal break.*
3. The pharmacist is considered directly and immediately available to patients during a meal break if patients are informed that they may request a pharmacist contact them at their earliest convenience after the meal break and if the pharmacist is available for consultation for emergency matters.
4. Registered pharmacy technicians may remain in the pharmacy during a pharmacist's meal break and are considered under the direct and personal supervision of the pharmacist if the pharmacist is available on the premises during the meal break to respond to questions by the technicians, and if at the end of the meal break, the pharmacist certifies all prescriptions prepared by the registered pharmacy technicians during the meal break.
5. Only prescriptions with a final certification by the pharmacist may be delivered.

STUDY TIP: Remember, a pharmacist may take up to a 30-minute meal break but cannot leave the premises. The pharmacy is not considered closed during this time, and registered pharmacy technicians may remain in the pharmacy.

E. Generic Substitution and Substitution of Biosimilar Products (§ 465.025, 465.0251, and 465.0252)
1. Pharmacists must substitute a generic equivalent unless requested otherwise by the purchaser if the drug is on the pharmacy's positive formulary.
Note: Substitution is mandatory if the product is on a pharmacy's positive formulary. All community pharmacies are required to have a positive formulary. See 3. below
2. Prohibition of Substitution
   a. For written prescriptions, a prescriber may prohibit substitution by writing the words "MEDICALLY NECESSARY" in his or her own handwriting on the prescription.
   b. For verbal prescriptions, a prescriber may prohibit substitution by expressly indicating to the pharmacist that the brand name drug prescribed is medically necessary.
   c. For electronic prescriptions, a prescriber may prohibit substitution by making an overt act to indicate that the brand name drug prescribed is medically necessary.

3. Positive Formulary (Rule 6416-27.520)
   a. Each community pharmacy shall develop a formulary of generic and brand name drugs which if substituted would not pose a threat to the health and safety of patients.
   b. The formulary shall be made available to the public, the Board of Pharmacy, or any physician requesting it.
4. Negative Formulary (Rule 64B16-27.500)
   a. The Board of Pharmacy and the Board of Medicine shall develop a formulary of drugs that demonstrate clinically significant biological or therapeutic inequivalence which may not be substituted.
   b. The Board of Pharmacy and the Board of Medicine must remove a drug from the Negative Formulary if every commercially marketed equivalent of the drug has an "A" rating in the FDA Orange Book.
   c. A pharmacist may not substitute a generic drug for a prescribed brand name drug if it is listed on the Negative Formulary.
   d. If a drug is prescribed that is on the Negative Formulary, but no brand name is specified, a pharmacist must dispense a product that has an approved New Drug Application or Abbreviated New Drug Application to market the drug.
      Note: In this case, whichever brand is dispensed should also be used for any refills.
   e. Current drugs on the negative drug formulary are:
      (1) Digitoxin
      (2) Conjugated Estrogens
      (3) Dicumarol
      (4) Chlorpromazine (solid oral dosage forms)
      (5) Theophylline (controlled release)
      (6) Pancrelipsase (oral dosage forms)

STUDY TIP: Even though many of the drugs on the Negative Formulary are not used much anymore, it is such a unique law to Florida that it is recommended that candidates memorize this list.

5. Every community pharmacy shall publicly display in a prominent place with a clear and unobstructed view, at or near the place where prescriptions are dispensed, a sign

in block letters not less than 1 in. in height, which reads: "CONSULT YOUR PHARMACIST CONCERNING THE AVAILABILITY OF A LESS EXPENSIVE GENERICALLY EQUIVALENT DRUG AND THE REQUIREMENTS OF FLORIDA LAW."

6. Notification of Substitution (§ 465.0244 and Rule 64B16-27.530)
   a. Prior to delivery of a prescription, a pharmacist must notify a patient of any generic substitution, the amount of the price difference, and the patient's right to refuse the substitution.
   b. This information must be communicated at a meaningful time to allow the patient to make an informed choice regarding substitution.
   c. The method of communication may be determined by the pharmacist.
   d. A pharmacist must also inform a patient if their cost-sharing obligation (i.e., copay) exceeds the retail price of the prescription if they paid cash.
7. Substitution of Interchangeable Biological Products (§ 465.0252)
   a. A pharmacist may only dispense a substitute biological product if the FDA has determined that the product is biosimilar and interchangeable for the prescribed biological product.
   Note: These determinations can be found in the FDA Purple Book. See Chapter 1
   b. The Board is required to maintain a list of current biological products that FDA has determined are biosimilar and interchangeable.
   Note: While there are several biosimilar products on the market (such as adalimumab, bevacizumab, and epoetin alfa), as of the date of publication of this book, FDA has not designated any of them as interchangeable.

F. Transfers and Common Database (§§ 465.026, 465.0266, and Rules 64B16-27.105, 64B16-28.451)
   1. Transfers—A pharmacist may fill or refill a valid prescription on file in a pharmacy in this state or another state that has been transferred from one pharmacy to another by any means, including electronically, under the following conditions:

- **a.** Prior to transfer, the pharmacist must either verbally or electronically:
  - **(1)** Advise the patient that the prescription on file at the other pharmacy must be cancelled;
  - **(2)** Determine that the prescription is valid and may be filled or refilled;
  - **(3)** Notify the pharmacist or pharmacy where the prescription is on file that the prescription must be cancelled;
  - **(4)** Record in writing or electronically the prescription information, the name of the pharmacy transferred from, the prescription number, the name of the drug, the original amount dispensed, the date of original dispensing, and the number of remaining authorized refills; and
  - **(5)** Obtain the consent of the prescriber when the pharmacist deems it necessary using his or her professional judgment.
- **b.** Requirements—When receiving a transfer request, the pharmacist must:
  - **(1)** Transfer the information required in a. (4) above to the pharmacist;
  - **(2)** Record on the prescription or electronically record the name of the requesting pharmacy, the name of the pharmacist, and the date of the request; and
  - **(3)** Cancel the prescription by electronic means or by writing the word "void" on the prescription record.
- **c.** If a transferred prescription is not dispensed within a reasonable time, the pharmacist shall notify the transferring pharmacy, which serves to revalidate the cancelled prescription.
- **d.** Electronic transfers of prescriptions are permitted regardless of whether the transferor or transferee pharmacy is open for business.

STUDY TIP: Recall that DEA only allows transfer of refills and not of original prescriptions for controlled substances, although by policy, they allow original prescriptions to be transferred if they are electronic prescriptions for controlled substances. *See Chapter 2*

2. Common Database
   a. Pharmacies that are under common ownership or utilize a common database may dispense a prescription in the common database and such a dispensing is NOT considered a transfer.
   b. See Specific requirements in § 465.0266 and Rule 64B16-28.451.

STUDY TIP: Be sure you understand the difference between a transfer and dispensing from a common database.

G. Central Fill Rules Specific to Community Pharmacy. *See II. H. above for general rules*
   1. A community central fill pharmacy may deliver non-controlled medications for an originating pharmacy directly to a patient if the pharmacies have a pharmacist available 40 hours a week, either in person or via two-way communication technology (telephone, etc.), and a toll-free number to provide counseling.
   2. A central fill pharmacy (including a community central fill pharmacy) may not deliver controlled substances directly to a patient.
   3. When a central fill pharmacy delivers a filled prescription directly to a patient, it is not considered dispensing.
   Note: It is treated more like the central fill pharmacy is delivering the prescription on behalf of the originating pharmacy.
   4. A community pharmacy that acts only as a central fill pharmacy and notifies the Board is exempt from requirements for a patient counseling area (Rule 64B16-28.1035), signage requirements (Rule 64B16-28.109(1)), and operating hours (Rule 64B16-28.1081).
H. Emergency Prescription Refill (§ 465.0275)
   Note: This law is not specific to community pharmacies but is placed here because it is usually done in a community pharmacy.
   1. In the event a pharmacist receives a request for a prescription refill and the pharmacist is unable to readily obtain refill authorization from the prescriber, the pharmacist may dispense:
      a. A onetime emergency refill of up to a 72-hour supply of the prescribed medication; or
      b. A onetime emergency refill of one vial of insulin.

2. If the Governor issues an emergency order or proclamation of a state of emergency, the pharmacist may dispense up to a 30-day supply in the area or counties affected by the order or proclamation, provided that:
   a. The prescription is not for a Schedule II controlled substance; and
   b. The medication is essential to the maintenance of life or to the continuation of therapy in a chronic condition.
3. Other Requirements:
   a. The emergency refill may be provided by a pharmacist if, in the pharmacist's professional judgment, the interruption of therapy might reasonably produce undesirable health consequences or may cause physical or mental discomfort.
   b. The dispensing pharmacist creates a written order containing all of the information required on a prescription and signs that order.
   c. The dispensing pharmacist notifies the prescriber of the emergency dispensing within a reasonable time after such dispensing.

STUDY TIP: Florida allows emergency refills for both non-controlled drugs and Schedule III–V controlled substances. Because DEA is silent on emergency refills, it is advisable to answer a question on emergency refills based on the Florida law.

I. OBRA '90—Patient Records, DUR, and Counseling
   Note: These rules apply to all pharmacies that dispense prescriptions.
   1. Requirement for Patient Record (Rule 64B16-27.800)
      a. All pharmacies must have a patient record system that provides for immediate retrieval of information necessary for the dispensing pharmacist to identify previously dispensed drugs.
      b. The pharmacist must ensure that a reasonable effort is made to obtain, record, and maintain the following information:
         (1) Name of the patient;
         (2) Address and telephone number of the patient;
         (3) Age or date of birth of the patient;
         (4) Patient's gender;

    (5) A list of new and refill prescriptions obtained by the patient at the pharmacy during the previous four years; and
    (6) Pharmacist's comments relevant to patient's drug therapy.

STUDY TIP: The original federal rules under OBRA '90 state that the pharmacist's comments would be considered reasonable if an impartial observer could review the documentation and understand what has occurred in the past, including what the pharmacist told the patient, information discovered about the patient, and what the pharmacist thought of the patient's drug therapy. Although not specifically mentioned in the Florida laws and rules, this should be considered a requirement for documentation of patient counseling for purposes of the MPJE.

---

   c. The pharmacist shall ensure that a reasonable effort is made to obtain from the patient and shall record any known allergies, drug reactions, idiosyncrasies, and chronic conditions or disease states and the identity of any other drugs, including OTC drugs or devices used by the patient.
   d. Patient records shall be maintained for a period not less than 4 years from the date of the last entry in the profile record.
 2. Prospective Drug Use Review (Rule 64B16-27.810)
   a. A pharmacist shall review the patient record and each new and refill prescription presented for dispensing in order to promote therapeutic appropriateness by identifying:
    (1) Overutilization or underutilization;
    (2) Therapeutic duplication;
    (3) Drug-disease contraindications;
    (4) Drug-drug interactions;
    (5) Incorrect drug dosage or duration of treatment;
    (6) Drug-allergy interactions; and
    (7) Clinical abuse/misuse.
   b. Upon recognizing any of the above, the pharmacist shall take appropriate steps to avoid or resolve the potential problems which shall, if necessary, include consultation with the prescriber.

3. Patient Counseling and Patient Consultation Area (Rules 64B16-27.820 and 64B16-28.1035)
   a. Community pharmacies must have a private consultation area designated with a sign.
   b. Upon receipt of a new or refill prescription, a pharmacist shall ensure that a verbal and printed offer to counsel is made to the patient or patient's agent when present.

STUDY TIP: Florida does not have mandatory patient counseling, but requires an offer to counsel (both written and printed) for both new and refill prescriptions.

   c. If a prescription is delivered outside of the pharmacy, the offer shall be in writing and shall provide for toll-free telephone access to the pharmacist.
   d. If the patient does not refuse counseling, the pharmacist shall review the patient's record and discuss matters which will enhance or optimize drug therapy.
   e. Elements of counseling are up to the professional judgment of the pharmacist, but may include the following:
      (1) Name and description of the drug;
      (2) Dosage form, dose, route of administration, and duration of therapy;
      (3) Intended use of the drug and expected action;
      (4) Special directions and precautions for preparation, administration, and use;
      (5) Common severe side effects or adverse effects or interactions and therapeutic contraindications that may be encountered, including their avoidance, and the action required if they occur;
      (6) Techniques for self-monitoring drug therapy;
      (7) Proper storage;
      (8) Prescription refill information;
      (9) Action to be taken in the event of a missed dose; and
      (10) Pharmacist comments relevant to drug therapy.
   f. Counseling is not required for inpatients of a hospital or institution where licensed healthcare practitioners are authorized to administer drugs (nursing homes, etc.).
   g. Counseling is not required when patient or patient's agent refuses such consultation.

J. Outpatient Dispensing Using an Automated Pharmacy System (§ 465.0235(2))
   1. A community pharmacy may provide pharmacy services for outpatient dispensing through the use of an automated pharmacy system that need not be located at the same location as the community pharmacy if:
      a. The automated pharmacy system is under the supervision and control of the community pharmacy.
      b. The automated pharmacy system is housed in an indoor environment area and in a location to increase patients' access to their prescriptions, including, but not limited to, medical facilities or places of business where essential goods and commodities are sold or large employer workplaces or locations where access to a community pharmacy is limited.
      c. The community pharmacy providing services through the automated pharmacy system notifies the board of the location of the automated pharmacy system and any changes in such location.
      d. The automated pharmacy system has a mechanism that provides live, real-time patient counseling by a pharmacist licensed in this state before the dispensing of any medicinal drug.
      e. The automated pharmacy system does not contain or dispense any controlled substance.
      f. The community pharmacy maintains a record of the medicinal drugs dispensed, including the identity of the pharmacist responsible for verifying the accuracy of the dosage and directions and providing patient counseling.
      g. The automated pharmacy system ensures the confidentiality of personal health information.
   2. Policies and Procedures
      a. The community pharmacy must maintain written policies and procedures to ensure the proper, safe, and secure functioning of the automated pharmacy system.
      b. The community pharmacy shall annually review the policies and procedures and maintain a record of such policies and procedures for a minimum of 4 years.
      c. The policies and procedures must, at a minimum, address all of the following:

(1) Maintaining the automated pharmacy system and any accompanying electronic verification process in good working order.
(2) Ensuring the integrity of the automated pharmacy system's drug identifier database and its ability to identify the person responsible for making database entries.
(3) Ensuring the accurate filling, stocking, restocking, and verification of the automated pharmacy system.
(4) Ensuring the sanitary operation of the automated pharmacy system and the prevention of cross-contamination of cells, cartridges, containers, cassettes, or packages.
(5) Testing the accuracy of the automated pharmacy system and any accompanying electronic verification process. The automated pharmacy system and accompanying electronic verification process must, at a minimum, be tested before the first use of the system, upon restarting the system, and after a modification of the system or electronic verification process which alters the filling, stocking, or restocking of the system or the electronic verification process.
(6) Training of persons authorized to access, stock, restock, or use the system.
(7) Conducting routine and preventative maintenance of the automated pharmacy system, including calibration of the system, if applicable.
(8) Removing expired, adulterated, misbranded, or recalled medicinal drugs from the automated pharmacy system.
(9) Preventing unauthorized persons from accessing the automated pharmacy system, including assigning, discontinuing, or modifying security access.
(10) Identifying and recording persons responsible for filling, stocking, and restocking the automated pharmacy system.
(11) Ensuring compliance with state and federal law, including, but not limited to, all applicable labeling, storage, and security requirements.
(12) Maintaining an ongoing quality assurance program that monitors and records performance of the

automated pharmacy system and any accompanying electronic verification process to ensure proper and accurate functioning, including tracking and documenting system errors.

K. Requirements for Use of an Automated Pharmacy System by a Community Pharmacy (Rule 64B16-28.141)
Note: At the time of publication of this book, the Board of Pharmacy had not yet made modifications to this rule to address using an automated system in locations separate from the pharmacy as permitted by the new law outlined in J. above.

1. An automated pharmacy system is a mechanical system that performs operations or activities, other than compounding or administration, relative to the storage, packaging, dispensing, or distribution of medication, and which collects, controls, and maintains all transaction information.
2. Location
   a. An automated pharmacy system may be located in the prescription department, adjacent to the prescription department, or on the establishment of the licensed pharmacy.
   b. If it is not located within the prescription department, it must have displayed on the system the name, address, contact information, and permit number of the community pharmacy that is responsible for its operation.
3. Requirements to be outlined in a policy and procedure manual:
   a. A method to ensure security of the system to prevent unauthorized access;
   b. A process of filling and stocking the system with drugs, including an electronic or hard-copy record of medication filled into the system with product identification, lot number, and expiration date;
   c. A method of identifying all registered pharmacy interns or registered pharmacy technicians involved in the dispensing process;
   d. Compliance with a continuous quality improvement program;
   e. A method to ensure patient confidentiality; and
   f. A process to enable the prescription department manager or designee to revoke, add, or change access at any time.

4. Additional Requirements:
   a. The system must maintain readily retrievable electronic records to identify all individuals involved in the dispensing of a prescription.
   b. The system must be able to comply with product recalls.
5. A prescription dispensed by an automated pharmacy system that meets the requirement of the rule is deemed to have been certified by the pharmacist.
6. Additional requirements apply to patient-accessed automated pharmacy systems. *See rule for details*

L. Closing a Pharmacy; Transfer of Files (Rule 64B16-28.202)
Note: This rule does not specify that it is only for community pharmacies, but it relates to prescription files, which are primarily seen in community pharmacies.
1. Prior to closing a pharmacy:
   a. Notification must be made in writing to the Board of Pharmacy indicating the date of closure and advising the Board which permittee is to receive the prescription files.
   b. The pharmacy permit must be returned to the Board.
2. On the day of closing the pharmacy must:
   a. Physically deliver the prescription files to a pharmacy within a reasonable proximity of the pharmacy closing.
   b. Affix a sign on the front entrance of the pharmacy advising the public of the new location of the prescription files or otherwise provide a means to advise the public of the new location.
3. A pharmacy receiving custody of prescription files from another pharmacy shall maintain the delivered prescription files separately.
4. The Board of Pharmacy's website includes the following instructions for closing a pharmacy, which are more specific than the rule.
   a. Please notify the board as soon as possible of the anticipated closing date. This notice must be submitted in writing and must contain the following information:
      (1) Date of closing.
      (2) The names and addresses of the persons who shall have custody of the prescription files, and the controlled drug inventory records of the pharmacy to be closed.

(3) The names and addresses of any persons who will acquire any of the legend drugs from the pharmacy to be closed.
- **b.** No later than ten days after the pharmacy has been closed, the pharmacy permit must be returned to the board office, and the permittee shall file a written report with the board office containing all of the following information:
  - **(1)** Confirmation that a sign has been posted outside of the closed establishment indicating the name and address of the pharmacy where the prescription files have been transferred.
  - **(2)** Confirmation that all legend drugs have been transferred to an authorized person or destroyed. If transferred, provide the names of all persons to whom they were transferred.
  - **(3)** If controlled drugs were transferred, the report must indicate the names and addresses of the persons to whom they were transferred.
  - **(4)** Confirmation that DEA registration and all blank DEA 222 (order forms) were returned to the DEA Miami Regional Office.

M. Miscellaneous Laws and Rules Relating to Community Pharmacies
  1. Dispensing of Schedule II or III Controlled Substances (§ 465.0181)
     - **a.** Only community pharmacies (including limited community pharmacy permits) can dispense Schedule II or III controlled substance prescriptions.
     - **b.** This was put in place in the midst of the opioid crisis to eliminate most physician dispensing of these products.
     - **c.** There are some exceptions in the dispensing practitioner statute in the medical practice act in § 456.0266.
  2. Faxed Prescriptions (§ 465.035)
     Pharmacists may fill prescriptions from fax orders sent by the patient, but may not dispense the prescription until they have the original written prescription. *Note: This law was enacted prior to mandatory electronic prescriptions but would still apply if an exception to the mandatory electronic prescription applies.*

3. Unclaimed Prescriptions (Rule 64B16-28.1191)
   Unclaimed prescriptions may be retained by a pharmacy and be reused for a period of one year from the date of filling unless it has an earlier expiration date.
   Note: This is for prescriptions that were filled but not picked up by patients. Because they never left control of the pharmacy, they are not considered a return of a dispensed drug. The Board also indicated in a declaratory statement that drugs that were shipped to a patient but not delivered have not been dispensed and may also be returned to stock. However, the pharmacist making the decision to return the drugs to stock of the pharmacy must exercise his or her professional judgment in deciding whether or not it is appropriate to return the drugs to stock in light of the conditions under which the drugs were stored prior to the return to the pharmacy.
4. Medicaid Audits and Pharmacy Audit Rights (§§ 465.188 and 465.1885)
   a. These two statutes provide pharmacies specific rights when being audited by Medicaid or an insurance company, third-party payor, a pharmacy benefit manager, or a similar entity.
   b. Since these provisions are not included in the MPJE Competencies, the details are not provided.

V. **Institutional Pharmacies**
   A. Rules Applicable to All Institutional Pharmacies
      1. Consultant Pharmacist of Record (Rule 64B16-28.501)
         a. All institutional pharmacy permits must have a licensed pharmacist designated as the consultant pharmacist of record.
         b. The Board of Pharmacy must be notified of a change in the consultant pharmacist of record within 10 days of the change.
         c. The consultant pharmacist of record must conduct a Drug Regiment Review, inspect the facility, and prepare a written report to be filed at the facility at least monthly.
         d. Remote access—a consultant pharmacist of record may access a facility or pharmacy's electronic database from outside the facility.
      2. Labeling of Drugs for Inpatient of a Nursing Home (Rule 64B16-28.502)

       a. Name and address of the pharmacy
       b. Name of the prescriber
       c. Name of the patient
       d. Date of original filling or refill date
       e. Prescription number
       f. Directions for use
       g. Name of the drug
       h. Quantity
       i. Transfer warning if it is a controlled substance

       Note: This is required labeling if using conventional dispensing bottles. See unit-dose labeling for alternative labeling.

3. Labeling of Repackaged or Unit-Dose Drugs
       a. Brand or generic name
       b. Strength
       c. Dosage form
       d. Name of manufacturer
       e. Expiration date
       f. Lot number (manufacturer's lot number or lot number assigned by the pharmacy)

STUDY TIP: When repackaged or unit-dose drugs are utilized in an institutional pharmacy, the patient-specific information does not have to appear on the individual label as long as the unit-dose system clearly indicates the name of the patient or resident, the prescription number or other means for identifying the medication order, the directions for use, and the name of the prescriber.

4. Prepackaging of Medications and Storage of Drugs (Rule 64B16-28.120(3) and (4))
       a. All prepackaging or unit-dose packaging of drugs must be done in accordance with procedures set up by the consultant pharmacist of record.

STUDY TIP: There is no specific Florida rule that addresses beyond-use dating for prepackaging or unit-dose packaging of solid oral dosage units (other than for customized medication packages), so it is likely that the general rule on beyond-use dates found in Rule 64B16-28.108(2)(h) of not greater than one year or the original expiration date, if that is less than one year, applies to drugs prepackaged in a pharmacy.

    b. Drugs stored in treatment areas must be accessible only to licensed staff (pharmacists, nurses, physicians, advanced practice registered nurses, physician assistants, respiratory and physical therapists, radiology technicians, registered pharmacy technicians, etc.) in accordance with their license, practice act, or to other personnel specifically authorized by the institution.

5. Return of Drugs in a Closed Drug Delivery System (Rule 64B16-28.118)
    a. A "closed drug delivery system" is a system in which the actual control of unit-dose or customized patient medication packages are maintained by the facility (Class I, Class II, Modified Class II, or Special ALF facilities) and not by the individual patient.
    b. In a closed drug delivery system, unused unit-dose or customized medication packages may be returned to the pharmacy for re-dispensing if each individual package is individually sealed and is clearly labeled with the name of the drug, dosage strength, manufacturer's control number, and expiration date.

STUDY TIP: The general rule is that once a drug has been dispensed to a patient, it cannot be returned to be re-dispensed. This exception is for closed-drug delivery systems only and is only for non-controlled drugs, as DEA does not permit this for controlled substances.

B. Transmission of Starter Dose Prescriptions for Patients in Class I or Modified Class II B Institutional Facilities (Rule 64B16-28.503)
  1. Definitions
    a. "Vendor pharmacy" is a community pharmacy or Special Closed Door Pharmacy which has a contract to dispense drugs to a patient in a facility holding a Class I Institutional Pharmacy or Modified Class II B permit.
    b. "Starter dose pharmacy" is a pharmacy that dispenses a medicinal drug pursuant to a starter dose prescription for a patient served by the vendor pharmacy.
    c. "Starter dose prescription" is a prescription transmitted by a vendor pharmacy to a starter dose pharmacy for the purpose of initiating drug therapy for a patient in a facility serviced by the vendor pharmacy.

2. A vendor pharmacy may transmit a starter dose prescription, excluding a controlled substance prescription, to a starter dose pharmacy if the vendor pharmacy:
   a. Has written authorization from the facility to use a starter dose pharmacy;
   b. Has written authorization from the prescriber, directly or via facility agreement, to act as the prescriber's agent to transmit the starter dose prescription;
   c. Has a valid prescription from the prescriber prior to transmitting the starter dose prescription;
   d. Maintains a record of each starter dose prescription; and
   e. Maintains a policy and procedure manual that references starter dose prescription.

STUDY TIP: This allows a pharmacy servicing a facility such as a nursing home to get a new prescription to a patient, quickly utilizing a closer, local pharmacy to provide the initial dose or doses.

C. Class II and Class III Institutional Pharmacy Laws and Rules
   1. Emergency Room Dispensing (§ 465.019(4) and Rule 64B16-28.6021)
      a. An individual licensed to prescribe medicinal drugs in this state may dispense up to a 24-hour supply of a medicinal drug to any patient of an emergency department of a hospital that operates a Class II or Class III institutional pharmacy, provided that the physician treating the patient in such hospital's emergency department determines that the medicinal drug is warranted and that community pharmacy services are not readily accessible, geographically or otherwise, to the patient.
      b. The following records of prescribing and dispensing must be created by the prescriber/dispenser and be maintained by the consultant pharmacist of record for the facility:
         (1) Patient name and address
         (2) Drug and strength prescribed/dispensed
         (3) Quantity prescribed/dispensed
         (4) Directions for use
         (5) Name of prescriber/dispenser
         (6) Prescriber DEA number if applicable
         (7) Reason community pharmacy services were not readily accessible

      c. Prescription container must meet all labeling requirements.
 2. Security (Rule 64B16-28.604)
      a. The pharmacy department in a hospital (Class II or Class III permit) shall be considered closed and shall be secured to prevent access when a Florida licensed pharmacist is not present and on duty.
      b. No person other than a Florida licensed pharmacist shall enter except as permitted by FPA § 465.019(2)(b) and Rule 64B16-28.602.

STUDY TIP: You have to look at two other sections to understand what this rule is saying, but the statute and rule state that when the pharmacy department is closed, a single dose may be obtained under the supervision of a physician or charge nurse. This implies that a nurse or physician could enter the pharmacy to obtain a single dose, but not other persons.

 3. Automated Distribution and Packaging (Rule 64B16-28.605)
      a. This rule provides requirements for using robotic, mechanical, or computerized devices designed to either distribute medications in a healthcare facility (decentralized automated distribution system such as Pyxis machines) or package medications for final distribution by a pharmacist (centralized automated distribution system).
      b. The consultant pharmacist of record is responsible for:
         (1) Maintaining a record of each transaction or operation;
         (2) Controlling access to the system;
         (3) Maintaining policies and procedures for operation, training, etc.;
         (4) Security;
         (5) Assuring that a patient receives the pharmacy services in a timely manner;
         (6) Assuring that the system maintains the integrity of information and protects patient confidentiality;
         (7) Establishing a comprehensive quality assurance program;
         (8) Establishing a procedure for stocking or restocking the system; and
         (9) Ensuring compliance with all packaging and labeling requirements.

c. A pharmacist must perform prospective drug use review and approve each medication order prior to administration except for an override medication, a low-risk override medication, or a physician-controlled medication.
   (1) An override medication is a single dose of a medication that may be removed from a decentralized automated medication system prior to pharmacist review because a practitioner has determined that the clinical status of the patient would be significantly compromised by delay.
   (2) A low-risk override medication is a medication determined to have a low risk of drug allergy, drug interaction, dosing error, or adverse patient outcome.
   (3) A physician-controlled medication is a medication distributed in an environment where a practitioner controls the order, preparation, and administration of the medication.
   Note: Examples would be emergency rooms, operating rooms, recovery rooms, cath labs, etc.
d. For override medications, a pharmacist shall perform a retrospective drug use review.
e. Decentralized automated medication systems may be restocked by a pharmacist, a registered pharmacy intern, or a registered pharmacy technician.
   (1) A pharmacist must conduct a daily audit of medications placed or to be placed into an automated medication system using random sampling; or
   (2) The system may use bar code verification, electronic verification, or similar verification processes to assure correct selection of medication placed or to be placed into an automated medication system.
f. A decentralized medication system that contains controlled substances shall not allow simultaneous access to multiple drugs, drug strengths, or dosage forms of controlled substances. *Note: Some automated systems use open or matrix drawers that, when opened, allow access to more than one drug.*
g. Centralized automated medication—A pharmacist may distribute patient-specific medications within a facility without checking each individual medication selected or packaged by the system if:

(1) The initial medication order has been reviewed and approved by a pharmacist;
(2) The medication is distributed for subsequent administration; and
(3) A bar code verification, electronic verification, or similar verification process is utilized to assure correct selection of medication placed or to be placed into the automated medication system.
  h. A Quality Assurance Program is required for all automated medication systems.
  i. Records must be maintained as follows:
     (1) 60 days for daily audits (if applicable) and transactions for all non-controlled substances; and
     (2) 4 years for any report or analysis that is part of the quality assurance program; any report or database related to access to the system or any change in access to the system, or medication in the system, and transaction records for all controlled substances.
4. Remote Medication Order Processing (Rule 64B16-28.606)
   Note: This rule also applies to Special Pharmacy Permits servicing Class I, Class II, Modified Class II, Class III, and Special ALF permitted facilities.
   a. Remote medication order processing includes any of the following activities:
      (1) Receiving, interpreting, or clarifying medication orders;
      (2) Entering or transferring medication order data;
      (3) Performing prospective drug use review;
      (4) Obtaining substitution authorizations;
      (5) Interpreting and acting on clinical data;
      (6) Performing therapeutic interventions;
      (7) Providing drug information;
      (8) Authorizing the release of medication for administration.
   b. Remote medication order processing is permitted if the pharmacist performing the activities has access to sufficient patient information necessary to perform prospective drug use review and approval of medication orders.
   c. All pharmacists participating in remote medication order processing shall be Florida licensed pharmacists.

d. A policy and procedure manual is required with specific information. *See rule for details*
   e. Records must be maintained that identify the name, initials, or identification code of each person who performed a processing function for every medication order.
D. Emergency Medication Kits in Nursing Homes
   1. Pharmacies serving nursing homes generally provide patient-specific medication often utilizing special packaging for unit-dose or customized patient medication packages.
   2. Nursing homes are required to also have an Emergency Medication Kit containing a limited supply of medications for use during an emergency that are not labeled for a specific patient.
   3. Florida law does not specify the types or quantity of drugs that may be maintained in an Emergency Medication Kit.
   4. The contents of the Emergency Medication Kit must be determined by the facility's medical director, director of nursing, and consultant pharmacist and may include controlled substances.

STUDY TIP: An Emergency Medication Kit in a nursing home is one of the rare exceptions where DEA allows non-dispensed (or bulk) controlled substances to be stored at a location that does not have a DEA registration.

   5. An inventory of the contents of the Emergency Medication Kit must be attached to the outside of the kit, which must include the earliest expiration date of the kit drugs. If the seal is broken, the kit must be restocked and resealed the next business day after use.
E. Automated Pharmacy Systems in Long Term Care, Hospice, and Correctional Facilities (§ 465.0235 and Rule 64B16-28.607)
   Note: New legislation effective July 1, 2020, expanded § 465.0235 to also allow use of automated pharmacy systems in outpatient settings. At the time of publication of this book, the Board of Pharmacy had not yet adopted rules to implement this legislation. Since the use in outpatient locations is from a community pharmacy, that change is located under the "Community Pharmacy" section of this book.
   1. A provider pharmacy may provide pharmacy services to a long-term care facility, hospice, or correctional facility using an automated pharmacy system.

2. The drugs stored in an automated pharmacy system at such facilities shall be owned by the provider pharmacy.
3. The drugs in an automated pharmacy system at such facilities are part of the inventory of the provider pharmacy and not part of the inventory of any other pharmacy permit for the facility.
4. A provider pharmacy shall have policies and procedures to ensure adequate security.
5. Drugs may be removed from an automated pharmacy system for administration to a patient only after a prescription order has been received and approved by a pharmacist at the provider pharmacy. This does not apply if the automated pharmacy system is also being used as an Emergency Medication Kit.
6. A pharmacist at the provider pharmacy shall control all operations of the automated pharmacy system and approve release of the initial dose of a prescription or order. Subsequent doses may be released without additional approval.
7. Stocking of the automated pharmacy system at the facility shall be accomplished by a pharmacist or other licensed personnel unless the system uses removable pockets or drawers that can be filled at the provider pharmacy and uses bar code verification, electronic verification, or similar verification to assure that the cartridge or drawer is accurately loaded into the system.
8. If an automated pharmacy system stores controlled substances, a DEA registration is required.

STUDY TIP: Although DEA does not require a separate DEA registration at a nursing home that is storing controlled substances in an Emergency Medication Kit, if the nursing home is using an automated pharmacy system to dispense routine medication or as an Emergency Medication Kit, a separate DEA registration for the automated pharmacy system at the facility, in the name of the provider pharmacy, is required.

9. An automated medication system that contains controlled substances shall not allow simultaneous access to multiple drugs, drug strengths, or dosage forms of controlled substances.

F. Institutional Formularies and Therapeutic Substitution in Nursing Homes (F.S. §§ 400.143 and 465.025(9))
   1. Legislation effective July 1, 2020, authorizes nursing homes to implement an institutional formulary and for a pharmacist to therapeutically substitute medicinal drugs under the established formulary.

STUDY TIP: "Therapeutic substitution" is defined as the practice of replacing a nursing home facility resident's prescribed medicinal drug with another chemically different medicinal drug that is expected to have the same clinical effect. This is often done in hospitals, but this law permits the practice in nursing homes.

---

   2. The nursing home must:
      a. Establish a committee to develop the institutional formulary and written guidelines or procedures for such. The committee must consist of, at a minimum:
         (1) The facility's medical director;
         (2) The facility's director of nursing services; and
         (3) A consultant pharmacist.
      b. Establish methods and criteria for selecting and objectively evaluating all available pharmaceutical products that may be used as therapeutic substitutes.
      c. Establish policies and procedures for developing and maintaining the institutional formulary and for approving, disseminating, and notifying prescribers of the institutional formulary.
      d. Perform quarterly monitoring to ensure compliance with the policies and procedures and monitor the clinical outcomes in circumstances in which a therapeutic substitution has occurred.
   3. Additional Requirements
      a. A prescriber must authorize use of the institutional formulary for each patient.
      b. A nursing home facility must obtain the prescriber's approval for any subsequent change made to a nursing home facility's institutional formulary.
      c. A prescriber may opt out of the nursing home facility's institutional formulary with respect to a medicinal drug or class of medicinal drugs for any resident.

- d. A nursing home facility must notify the prescriber before each therapeutic substitution using a method of communication designated by the prescriber. A nursing home facility must document the therapeutic substitution in the resident's medical records.
- e. A prescriber may prevent a therapeutic substitution for a specific prescription by indicating "NO THERAPEUTIC SUBSTITUTION" on the prescription. If the prescription is provided orally, the prescriber must make an overt action to opt out of the therapeutic substitution.
- f. The nursing home facility must obtain informed consent from a resident or a resident's legal representative, or his or her designee, to the use of the institutional formulary for the resident. The nursing home facility must clearly inform the resident or the resident's legal representative, or his or her designee, of the right to refuse to participate in the use of the institutional formulary and may not take any adverse action against the resident who refuses to participate in the use of the institutional formulary.

4. A pharmacist may therapeutically substitute medicinal drugs in accordance with an institutional formulary established for the resident of a nursing home facility if the prescriber has agreed to the use of such institutional formulary for the patient. The pharmacist may not therapeutically substitute a medicinal drug pursuant to the facility's institutional formulary if the prescriber indicates on the prescription "NO THERAPEUTIC SUBSTITUTION" or overtly indicates that therapeutic substitution is prohibited.

VI. Nuclear Pharmacies and Nuclear Pharmacists
A. Nuclear Pharmacists (Rules 64B16-26.303 and 64B16-26.304)
1. Additional licensure requirements:
   a. At least 200 hours of formal didactic training from an accredited college of pharmacy or other recognized program on specified radiopharmaceutical topics.
   b. A radiopharmacy internship of at least 500 hours.
   c. If the didactic and experiential training have not been obtained within the last 7 years, the applicant must have been engaged in the practice of nuclear pharmacy in another jurisdiction for at least 1,080 hours in the last 7 years.

2. Additional continuing education requirements—24 additional hours on specified nuclear pharmacy topics.
3. Only a nuclear pharmacist may receive prescriptions for therapy (*Note: Should say "therapeutic"*) or blood product procedures in a permitted nuclear pharmacy.

STUDY TIP: In a nuclear pharmacy, a registered pharmacy technician may take an order for a diagnostic radiopharmaceutical, but not for a therapeutic or blood product procedure.

B. Nuclear Pharmacies (§ 465.0193)
   1. Definition—includes every location where radioactive drugs and chemicals within the classification of medicinal drugs are compounded, dispensed, stored, or sold. The term "nuclear pharmacy" does not include hospitals or the nuclear medicine facilities of such hospitals.
   2. Must have a prescription department manager.
   3. Must be secured from access by unauthorized personnel.
   4. Must have a secured radioactive storage and decay area.
   5. Must maintain accurate records of acquisition, inventory, distribution, and disposal of all radiopharmaceuticals.
   6. The name of the patient must be obtained prior to dispensing if the order is for therapeutic or blood product radiopharmaceuticals (as opposed to a diagnostic radiopharmaceutical).
   7. Diagnostic radiopharmaceuticals may be labeled "Physician's Use Only" if the name of the patient is readily retrievable from the physician upon demand.
   8. Immediate outside container must be labeled with:
      a. Name and address of the pharmacy
      b. Name of the prescriber
      c. Date of original filling
      d. Standard radiation symbol
      e. The words "Caution: Radioactive Material"
      f. Name of the procedure
      g. Prescription number
      h. Radionuclide and chemical form
      i. Amount of radioactivity and the calibration date and time
      j. Expiration date and time
      k. Volume if a liquid
      l. Number of items or weight if a solid

    m. Number of ampules or vials if a gas
    n. If for a Tc 99m product, the molybdenum 99 content to USP limits
    o. Name of the patient or "Physicians Use Only"
    p. Initials of the dispensing pharmacist
9. Immediate inner container must be labeled with:
    a. Standard radiation symbol
    b. The words "Caution: Radioactive Material"
    c. Radionuclide and chemical form
    d. Prescription number
10. Space and equipment requirements
    a. Area for storage, compounding, distribution, and disposal of radiopharmaceuticals shall be adequate to completely separate such radioactive pharmaceuticals from non-radioactive drugs.
    b. The hot lab, storage area, and compounding and dispensing area must be a minimum of 150 ft^2.
    c. Must have specified equipment. *See rule for details*

CHAPTER FIVE
USP Chapters and Compounding Laws and Rules

CHAPTER FIVE
USP Chapters and Compounding Laws and Rules

Special thanks to Patricia Kienle, RPh, MPA, BCSCP, FASHP, for providing the summaries of USP Chapters 797 and 800

I. **Introduction to USP Chapters**
   A. Legal Recognition
      1. USP sets standards for identity, strength, quality, and purity of medications. The standards are published in the United States Pharmacopeia-National Formulary (USP-NF) compendium.
      2. USP standards are recognized in the federal Food, Drug and Cosmetic Act (FDCA) and in various state laws and regulations. USP Chapters are considered *compendially applicable*, meaning they are enforceable under federal regulations when they are numbered under 1,000, and they are referenced in a General Notice, monograph, or another chapter numbered under 1,000.

STUDY TIP: When standards use the terms "must" or "shall," it is a requirement. When standards use the term "should," it is a recommendation.

   B. USP Components
      1. USP General Notices provide basic information for use of the standards, such as descriptions of dosage forms, temperature requirements, and other information.
      2. USP General Chapters contain established procedures, methods, and practices. USP 795, 797, and 800 are examples of General Chapters.
      3. USP Monographs contain specific information about a formulation or compound. The USP compendium contains almost 200 different compounding monographs.
      4. Monographs are more specific than General Chapters. General Chapters are more specific than General Notices. When information conflicts, the more specific document applies.
   C. Enforcement
      1. USP does not enforce the standards. Enforcement is accomplished by states and by accreditation organizations that incorporate the standards into their requirements.

2. The FDCA mandates use of USP standards for compounding.
3. When bulk drug substances (active pharmaceutical ingredients, or APIs) are used, those APIs must comply with the standards in a USP monograph (if one exists) and the applicable USP compounding standard (795 for nonsterile compounding or 797 for sterile compounding).
4. The 2013 Drug Quality and Security Act (DQSA) reaffirmed USP's authority over compounding in Section 503A. This Act distinguishes 503A entities (compounding pharmacies which supply patient-specific preparations) from 503B entities (outsourcing facilities which supply non-patient-specific preparations). Generally, 503A pharmacies are governed by state boards and follow USP compounding chapters. 503B outsourcing facilities are governed by the Food and Drug Administration (FDA) and must comply with more stringent current Good Manufacturing Practices (cGMPs).

D. Compounding
1. The FDA exempts compounding from the rigorous requirements for a new drug application, provided the compound is made by a licensed pharmacist or physician and complies with the USP Chapters on pharmacy compounding. The FDA also provides other guidance documents related to compounding.
2. States define compounding in their pharmacy rules and regulations.
3. Four General Chapters provide compounding information
   a. USP 795 Pharmaceutical Compounding—Nonsterile Preparations *Note: USP 795 has not been adopted by Florida and is not covered in this book.*
   b. USP 797 Pharmaceutical Compounding—Sterile Preparations
   c. USP 800 Hazardous Drug—Compounding in Healthcare Settings
      Note: USP 800 has not been adopted by Florida, but is covered in this book because it is specifically mentioned in the MPJE Competency Statements.
   d. USP 825 Radiopharmaceuticals—Preparation, Compounding, Dispensing, and Repackaging
      Note: USP 825 has not been adopted by Florida and is not covered in this book.

II. USP 797 Pharmaceutical Compounding—Sterile Preparations

Florida has adopted USP 797 with some modifications. USP Chapter 797 was last revised in 2008. A revision published in 2019 was intended to be official in December 2019 but has been delayed due to appeals to the Chapter. This information highlights the current official (2008) version, which Florida has adopted by rule.

A. Introduction and Scope

  1. Chapter 797 provides standards to prevent harm that could occur from microbial, chemical, or physical contamination; incorrect strength; or inappropriate quality of compounded sterile preparations (CSPs) for human and animal patients.

  2. Chapter 797 applies to all healthcare personnel who compound CNSPs and applies in all healthcare settings.

  3. CSPs include drugs and biologics such as injections, infusions, irrigations for wounds and body cavities, ophthalmics (including drops), tissue implants, baths and soaks for organs and tissues, aqueous bronchial and nasal inhalations, and other preparations intended to be sterile.

  4. Applicable state and federal laws and regulations concerning compounding must also be followed.

  5. If hazardous drugs are compounded, both USP 797 and USP 800 (*Hazardous Drugs—Handling in Healthcare Settings*) apply. The Occupational Safety and Health Administration (OSHA) and the National Institute for Occupational Safety and Health (NIOSH) have additional guidance concerning hazardous drugs.

  6. USP 797 has sections concerning the special requirements for preparation of allergen extracts and radiopharmaceuticals. The radiopharmaceutical information is now supplemented by a new USP Chapter: USP 825 *Radiopharmaceuticals—Preparation, Compounding, Dispensing, and Repackaging*.

STUDY TIP: Federal laws and regulations include those promulgated by agencies such as the Food and Drug Administration (FDA) and Centers for Medicare and Medicaid Services (CMS). State agencies include state boards of pharmacy and health. Accreditation organizations such as The Joint Commission and the Pharmacy Compounding Accreditation Board (PCAB) may also include USP standards in their requirements.

B. Categories of CSPs
   1. Immediate Use are those mixed outside of the facilities described in the chapter when the urgency does not permit mixing in a cleanroom suite or segregated compounding area (SCA). Immediate Use preparations are limited to simple transfer of not more than 3 sterile manufactured ingredients and not more than 2 entries into any one container.
   2. Low Risk CSPs are those mixed in a USP 797–compliant area as a single dose for one patient.
   3. Medium Risk CSPs are those mixed in a USP 797–compliant area as a batch for multiple patients or for one patient on multiple occasions, or more complex mixtures such as Total Parenteral Nutrition (TPN) solutions.
   4. High Risk CSPs are those mixed in a USP 797–compliant cleanroom suite with a nonsterile starting ingredient, or any risk level if mixed without complete garb as required.
   5. The risk levels are key elements in determining the beyond-use dates (BUDs) for sterile compounds.

STUDY TIP: Examples of types of risk levels include:
- Low—reconstituting a vial of cefazolin and placing it in a piggyback IV bag
- Medium—making a batch of ten antibiotic syringes
- High—mixing an alum irrigation from an Active Pharmaceutical Ingredient (API)

C. Responsibilities of Compounders
   1. The compounder is responsible for preparing CSPs that are accurately mixed, within 10% of labeled strength/potency (unless otherwise listed), and prepared with appropriate technique in proper facilities.
   2. Training
      a. Compounders must be trained and able to demonstrate competence for assigned activities.
      b. Initial training includes theoretical principles, practical skills including aseptic work practices, observation of expert compounders, and return demonstrations, and successful completion of written competences, hand hygiene and garbing, a gloved fingertip test without any contamination, and media fill tests.

    c. Requalifying training includes successful completion of written tests, media fill tests, and requalifying gloved fingertip tests. The media fill tests and requalifying glove fingertip tests must be done at least every 6 months if high-risk CSPs are mixed, or at least every 12 months if only low- and medium-risk CSPs are mixed.
    d. Media fill tests must mimic the most complex CSP mixed. A successful media fill test is one that shows no growth or cloudiness over the time period of the test.
    e. Gloved fingertip tests are done at initial training (to check for the ability to aseptically garb) and as a requalifying test at the same frequency as required for media fill tests.

STUDY TIP: Action Levels—the maximum number of microbial colony forming units (CFUs) allowed—are listed in USP 797 for the gloved fingertip test. Initially, the compounder needs to complete 3 sets (6 plates) with no growth to demonstrate the ability to repeatedly garb without contamination themselves. For requalification, the same test is done, but it is done following a media fill after other compounding. Only 1 set (2 plates) is required, and the number of CFUs cannot exceed 3 on both plates.

---

    f. All training must be documented.
D. Facilities
  1. The sterile compounding area must be properly designed with cleanable surfaces and should have a temperature under 20°C. No humidity requirement is listed in the 2008 version of USP 795, but the relative humidity should be under 60%. Some states have specific requirements.
  2. Primary Engineering Controls
    a. Primary Engineering Controls (PECs, informally called "hoods") are the devices in which CSPs are mixed.
    b. Laminar airflow workbenches (LAFWs) and biological safety cabinets (BSCs) are examples of traditional types of PECs.
    c. Compounding aseptic isolators (CAIs) and compounding aseptic containment isolators (CACIs) are examples of compounding isolators.
    d. PECs must meet specific criteria, including maintenance of an ISO 5 classification, have unidirectional airflow, and meet other requirements listed in USP 797.

STUDY TIP: ISO class is determined by the number of particles larger than 0.5 microns in a volume of air. The smaller the ISO number, the cleaner the air. PECs must be ISO 5 or cleaner. Anterooms that open into a negative pressure room and buffer rooms must be ISO 7 or cleaner. Anterooms that open only into positive pressure buffer rooms must be ISO 8 or cleaner.

3. Secondary Engineering Controls
   a. Secondary Engineering Controls (SECs, informally called the IV room or IV lab) are the rooms in which the PEC is placed.
   b. USP 797 details specific requirements including ISO classification, pressurization, airflow, and other characteristics.
   c. There are two types of SECs:
      (1) A cleanroom suite, consisting of a positive pressure anteroom and at least one buffer room. The anteroom must be positive pressure and must be at least ISO 7 if it opens into any negative pressure buffer room, or at least ISO 8 if it opens only into positive pressure buffer rooms. The buffer room must be at least ISO 7.
      (2) A segregated compounding area (SCA), which is an area designated for use for sterile compounding. It does not have to be a separate room, but that is preferred. A more complex containment segregated compounding area (C-SCA) is used for compounding hazardous drugs. (See the section on USP 800 for details.)

SEC	Minimum ISO Classification
Anteroom that opens only into positive pressure buffer room(s)	ISO 8
Anteroom that opens into one or more negative pressure room(s)	ISO 7
Positive pressure buffer room	ISO 7
Negative pressure buffer room	ISO 7
Segregated Compounding Area	Not required to be ISO-classified
Containment Segregated Compounding Area	Not required to be ISO-classified

STUDY TIP: Some states have specific requirements, including limitation of use of the area, minimum square footage, etc.

4. Pressure gradients between rooms in a sterile compounding suite minimize the possibility of microbial contamination.
   a. The buffer room (where the hood is placed) must be 0.020″ more positive than the anteroom.
   b. The anteroom must be 0.020″ more positive than the general area it opens into.
   c. There is no pressure gradient requirement for segregated compounding areas (SCAs).
   d. There is a negative pressure requirement for hazardous drug ("chemo") buffer rooms and C-SCAs. (See the chapter on USP 800 for details.)
5. Current (2008) USP 797 allows a clean-room that is a single room with an ante-area and a buffer area. A line dividing the two areas must be used to demonstrate airflow of 40 feet per minute from the buffer to ante-area. This design is not recommended and is unlikely to be allowed in the future.
6. Other Devices and Equipment
   a. The cleanroom suite or SCA must be designed to promote proper cleaning. Sinks, counters, passthroughs, refrigerators, and other equipment and devices must be suitable for use in the IV room, properly placed, and cleaned.
   b. Devices specifically designed for use in the PEC, such as automated compounding devices (ACDs) and repeater pumps, must be used according to manufacturer's instructions and only by compounders who have been assessed for competence.
7. Certification—PECs and SECs must be certified every 6 months by a qualified certification technician.

E. Hand Hygiene, Garb, and Personal Protective Equipment (PPE)
   1. Hand hygiene (i.e., hand washing) must be performed as detailed in the organization's policy. Hands and forearms must be washed with soap and water up to elbows for 30 seconds.
   2. Garb and PPE includes hair covers, face masks, gloves, gowns, and shoe covers. Additional PPE is required when compounding hazardous drugs (HDs).
   3. There is a specific order in which to don garb and perform hand hygiene:
      a. Don head and hair covers, masks, and shoe covers upon entry to the anteroom or SCA.

- **b.** Perform hand hygiene.
  - **c.** In an anteroom, step over into the clean side of the room.
  - **d.** Don gown.
  - **e.** Apply alcohol-based hand rub to hands and allow to dry.
  - **f.** Don sterile gloves.
- **F.** Standard Operating Procedures (SOPs) and Other Documentation
  - **1.** Standard Operating Procedures (SOPs)
    - **a.** The person in charge of compounding needs to establish and maintain adequate policies and procedures to ensure safe and reproducible CNSPs. SOPs should include details concerning facilities, equipment, personnel, receipt, storage, compounding, and other related elements.
    - **b.** When errors or other excursions occur, policies should guide the process to identify and correct the occurrence.
  - **2.** Master Formulation Records and Compounding Records are not required in the 2008 version of USP 797, but similar records are necessary. Some states require all the elements listed for the MFRs and CRs in USP 795 and in the proposed revision to USP 797 that was published in 2019. In any case, appropriate records should be developed and maintained, such as logs for batches of CSPs made.
- **G.** Compounding Technique
  - **1.** Aseptic technique is a core practice that must be mastered.
  - **2.** Maintaining sterility of critical sites is essential. Critical sites are areas such as vial septa, ports, needle hubs, and other surfaces at highest risk of exposure to contamination.
- **H.** Components
  - **1.** Ingredients must be obtained from reliable sources and stored according to manufacturer's information and applicable laws and regulations. When possible, ingredients meeting standards of the United States Pharmacopeia (USP), National Formulary (NF), or Food Chemicals Codex (FCC) should be used. Ingredients should be obtained from FDA-registered facilities when possible.
  - **2.** Ingredients must be stored appropriately and cannot be stored on the floor. Ingredients that have a manufacturer's or supplier's expiration date may be used through that date as long as the container is stored to avoid decomposition of the contents. If no expiration date is provided, the compounder must assign a date that is no longer than one year

from the date of receipt, unless testing proves it has retained the purity and quality required.
3. Active Pharmaceutical Ingredients (APIs) are the raw powders (sometimes called "bulk substances") used for compounding. Applicable Safety Data Sheets (SDSs) and other required documentation must be available for compounders.
4. APIs that are not USP or NF grade must be accompanied by a lot-specific Certificate of Analysis (COA).
5. Ingredients used for compounding CSPs for humans must not be those that have been withdrawn from the market for safety purposes.

I. Compounding Process
1. Most CSPs are mixed using only conventionally manufactured sterile components. The goal for sterile-to-sterile compounding is to maintain sterility.
2. High-risk CSPs are mixed using nonsterile starting ingredients. The goal for nonsterile-to-sterile compounding is to achieve sterility. Sterilization of the final CSP is achieved using terminal sterilization (such as in an autoclave using steam under pressure) or by filtration. Both methods require quality control measures to ensure they have performed as intended.
   a. Autoclaving is monitored using biological indicators.
   b. Filtration is checked by performing a bubble point test of the used filter to ensure its integrity.

STUDY TIP: Terminal sterilization is described in USP 797 as by use of an autoclave (steam under pressure) or dry heat. Filtration is not terminal sterilization.

3. High-risk CSPs (except those for inhalation or ophthalmic administration) that are made in groups of more than 25 units must also pass a bacterial endotoxin (pyrogen) test.
4. Components used for preparation of CSPs have limited in-use times:

Type of component	Allowable in-use time when opened in and maintained in ISO 5	Allowable in-use time when opened outside of or removed from ISO 5
Ampule	Use and discard remainder	Use and discard remainder
Single-dose vial	Up to 6 hours	Up to 1 hour
Multiple-dose vial	Up to 28 days (unless manufacturer's instructions differ)	Up to 28 day (unless manufacturer's instructions differ)

5. Assignment of Beyond-Use Dates (BUDs)
    a. The BUD is the date beyond which a CSP must not be used.

STUDY TIP: Expiration dates are provided by manufacturers for their products. BUDs are established by compounders for their preparations.

   b. BUDs for CSPs that do not have stability information for the specific formulation (including drug, diluent, container, and closure) must limit the BUDs assigned to the following:

Category	Stored at controlled room temperature	Stored under refrigeration	Stored frozen
Immediate Use	1 hour	Not applicable	Not applicable
Low Risk Made in an SCA	12 hours	12 hours	Not applicable
Low Risk	48 hours	14 days	45 days
Medium Risk	30 hours	9 days	45 days
High Risk	24 hours	3 days	45 days

   c. BUDs may be extended beyond the default dates above if stability studies of the formulation are conducted with appropriate results or if a USP monograph is followed exactly and contains a longer BUD.
   d. The BUD cannot be longer than the expiration date of any of its components.
6. Labeling
    Labels of CSPs must include the drug name and strength/concentration, total volume, BUD, route of administration, and storage conditions. Other information to support safe use, organizational policy, and state laws and regulations must be included as appropriate.

J. Dispensing the Final Preparation
    1. The compounder must check the final CSP prior to dispensing. Identification of the individual who checked the final CSP must be documented.
    2. Many CSPs require storage at refrigerator temperature if not immediately dispensed. Those CSPs that will be shipped to a location other than where they are compounded (e.g., to a patient's home) must have appropriate temperature control.

K. Cleaning the Compounding Areas
1. Solutions used must be appropriate for use in a clean-room and (if necessary) properly diluted. Many solutions have a *dwell time*, which is the time the solution needs to be wet and in contact with the surface in order to achieve its intended result (i.e., decontamination, cleaning, disinfection).
2. Cleaning PECs and SECs is done with a detergent. After cleaning, the PEC needs to have sterile 70% isopropyl alcohol applied to the surface of the PEC.
3. The PEC surface must be cleaned at the beginning of each shift, before each batch, every 30 minutes during compounding, after spills, and when surface contamination is known or suspected.
4. Floors, counters, and other easily cleanable surfaces (e.g., refrigerator handles, pass-through chambers) must be cleaned daily.
5. Storage shelving, walls, and ceilings must be cleaned at least monthly.
6. Only compounding personnel can clean the PECs, but some organizations allow others with documented competency to clean floors, walls, and ceilings.

L. Environmental Monitoring
1. Environmental monitoring consists of nonviable (e.g., temperature, pressure gradients, airflow) and viable (microbial contamination) elements.
2. Some nonviable parameters must be monitored daily by compounding personnel:
   a. Temperature of the compounding areas—should be 20°C or lower to minimize the risk of microbial contamination and for the comfort of the garbed compounder. If drugs are stored in the compounding area, the required temperature range for the drugs must be maintained.
   b. Pressure gradients between rooms. USP 797 requires minimum pressure gradients between rooms. Positive pressure rooms assist in preventing contamination entering the room, so are used for anterooms and nonhazardous buffer rooms. Negative pressure rooms assist in containing hazards, so are used for hazardous ("chemo") buffer rooms.

Between	Minimum pressure gradient required
Nonhazardous buffer room to anteroom	Buffer room must be at least 0.020" more positive than the anteroom
Hazardous buffer room to anteroom	Buffer room must be between 0.010 and 0.030" negative to anteroom
Anteroom to adjacent general area	Anteroom must be at least 0.020" more positive than general area
Segregated Compounding Area	No requirement
Containment Segregated Compounding Area to adjacent general area	C-SCA must be between 0.010 to 0.030" negative to adjacent area

    c. Combined ante/buffer rooms must have a displacement airflow of at least 40 feet per minute over the line of demarcation from the buffer area to the ante-area.

3. **Certification**

    Certification involves a qualified technician checking and ensuring that nonviable parameters listed in USP 797 (e.g., particle counts, airflow, proper pressurization, and other elements) are within manufacturer's and industry specifications. PECs must be certified every six months and after servicing. SECs must be certified every six months or when changes are made in the room that could affect the airflow.

4. **Viable Monitoring**

    a. The facilities in which low-, medium-, and high-risk CSPs are made must be monitored to ensure microbial (bacterial and fungal) contaminants are not present to a degree that could harm patients.

    b. Viable monitoring is accomplished with electronic air sampling and surface sampling.

    c. Electronic air sampling must be checked at least every 6 months. Surface sampling must be checked periodically. Most organizations have their certifiers perform this sampling. Many organizations supplement these semiannual checks with additional sampling. Facilities that mix only low- and medium-risk level CSPs must test for bacteria; facilities mixing high-risk level CSPs must test for bacteria and fungus. However, most organizations test for both bacteria and fungus even if they mix only low- and medium-risk CSPs.

    d. Action Levels based on the maximum number of CFUs allowed are listed in USP 797. If the action levels are exceeded or if trends are noted, the compounder needs to consult with a trained microbiologist to develop a remedial plan. Organisms exceeding the action level should be identified at least to the genus level. Highly pathogenic organisms (e.g., gram-negative rods, coagulase positive staphylococcus, molds, and yeasts) must be immediately remedied even if they do not exceed the action level.

ACTION LEVELS IN NUMBER OF COLONY FORMING UNITS (CFUS)

ISO Classification	Air Sample (per 1,000 liters of air)	Surface Sample (per plate)
ISO 5 (PECs)	>1	>3
ISO 7 (buffer rooms and anteroom opening into a negative pressure room)	>10	>5
ISO 8 (anteroom opening only into positive pressure buffer rooms)	>100	>100

M. Quality Control
1. A policy needs to be established to describe the elements of control that support safe sterile compounding.
2. The elements should be specific and measurable and identify the follow-up that would occur if excursions beyond stated limits occur.

III. USP 800 Hazardous Drugs—Compounding in Healthcare Settings
Note: USP Chapter 800 has not yet been adopted by the Florida Board of Pharmacy, but since it is listed in the MPJE Competency Statements, a brief summary is included below.
USP Chapter 800 became official on December 1, 2019.
A. Introduction and Scope
1. Chapter 800 details practice and quality standards for handling hazardous drugs (HDs) in various healthcare settings. The chapter discusses the handling of HDs from receipt to storage, compounding, dispensing, administration, and disposal of both nonsterile and sterile preparations. Included in the chapter is information on proper engineering controls and quality standards, personnel training, labeling, packaging, and transport and disposal of HDs, along with measures for spill control, documentation of all aspects of the handling of HDs, and medical surveillance.

2. Chapter 800 applies to all healthcare personnel and all entities who handle hazardous drugs. These personnel and entities include, but are not limited to, pharmacists, pharmacy technicians, pharmacies, physicians, nurses, hospital physician assistants, home healthcare workers, physician practice facilities, veterinarians, veterinary technicians, and veterinary hospitals and facilities. Entities that handle HDs must incorporate Chapter 800 standards into occupational safety standards.
3. The Occupational Safety and Health Administration (OSHA) includes hazardous drugs in their hazardous materials requirements, but does not include details of specific agents. Some states have additional state OSHA requirements.

B. List of Hazardous Drugs
1. The National Institute of Occupational Safety and Health (NIOSH) maintains a list of hazardous drugs (HDs) used in healthcare. This list is updated approximately every two years. Chapter 800 requires any entity that stores, compounds, prepares, transports, or administers hazardous drugs to maintain a list of HDs used in the entity and to review the list at least every 12 months and update whenever a new agent or dosage form is used. Newly marketed HDs or dosage forms should be reviewed against the entity's list.

STUDY TIP: The NIOSH list is split into tables. Table 1 includes antineoplastic drugs that must be handled with all containment and work practices listed in USP 800. Other drugs may be exempted by organizational policy in an assessment of risk if alternative strategies to protect personnel are identified and implemented.

2. The NIOSH list comprises drugs that are hazardous to healthcare workers. These are drugs that are carcinogens, genotoxins, teratogens, reproductive toxins, or cause organ toxicity at low doses. This is a different situation than hazardous materials defined by the Environmental Protection Agency (EPA), which are hazardous to the environment. A few hazardous drugs are listed on both lists.

STUDY TIP: NIOSH hazardous drugs are those that are hazardous to healthcare workers due to the potential of inadvertent personal contamination. EPA hazardous materials, some of which are drugs, are hazardous to the environment.

3. Some dosage forms of drugs defined as hazardous drugs may not pose a substantial risk of direct occupational exposure to healthcare workers. However, particulate matter from tablets, capsules, and/or packaging materials could present an exposure risk if it contacts skin or mucous membranes. Facilities using hazardous drugs must perform an assessment of risk at least annually to determine if new or alternate containment strategies need to be employed to mitigate risks for exposure from HDs.

STUDY TIP: Not all hazardous drugs have to be handled the same way. Hazardous drugs that will only be counted or packaged may not require all of the containment and/or work practices that an antineoplastic that must be compounded needs.

4. Unintentional exposures to hazardous drugs have been documented. These include transdermal and transmucosal absorption, injection, and ingestion. Containers of HDs have been shown to be contaminated upon arrival to their intended destination. Accidental exposure is also possible for individuals handling body fluids; deactivating, decontaminating, or disinfecting areas contaminated with HDs; and/or contacting HD residue on drug containers, work surfaces, etc.

C. Responsibilities of Personnel Handling Hazardous Drugs
   1. The chapter requires that each entity have a "Designated Person" to be responsible for developing and implementing HD handling procedures. This individual must be properly trained and qualified to oversee entity compliance with the chapter and applicable state and federal laws and regulations and to ensure competency of all individuals who may come into contact with HDs.

STUDY TIP: USP does not require the Designated Person to be a pharmacist, but some states may require that. The Designated Person does not need to be a manager, and that person may have responsibility for more than one location.

   2. All persons involved in the handling of HDs must have a fundamental understanding of practices and precautions and of the evaluation of procedures to ensure the safety and

quality of the final HD product or preparation to minimize the risk of harm to the intended patient.

D. Facilities and Engineering Controls
1. At each stage of the handling of HDs there must be conditions and policies in place to promote safety for patients, workers, and the environment.
2. Signs must be placed at entrances to HD handling areas. Access to these areas of a facility should be limited only to properly trained and authorized personnel.
3. The chapter requires that there be designated areas for receiving and unpacking HDs, for storing HDs, and for compounding of nonsterile and sterile preparations.
4. Certain areas must have a negative pressure gradient with respect to surrounding areas of the facilities to reduce the risk of contaminating areas where non-HD-authorized individuals work. These negative-pressure areas should have an uninterrupted power source in the event of a loss of power to the facility.

E. Receipt of HDs
1. According to Chapter 800, all HDs and all hazardous drug active pharmaceutical ingredients (HD-APIs) must be removed from shipping containers in an area that is negative pressure or neutral pressure relative to the surrounding areas. General receiving areas are acceptable as long as they are not positive pressure areas.
2. In addition, shipping cartons containing HDs and/or HD-APIs must not be opened in sterile compounding or positive pressure areas.

F. Storage of HDs
1. HDs must be stored in areas that can prevent or contain spillage or breakage of a container if it falls. However, HDs must not be stored on the floor.
2. Antineoplastic HDs in NIOSH Table 1 that will be compounded to make the final preparation and Active Pharmaceutical Ingredients (API) of any NIOSH HDs must be stored in an area away from non-HDs to prevent contamination or personnel exposure.
3. The room for storage of NIOSH Table 1 antineoplastic HDs that will be compounded and HD-APIs must be vented to the exterior of the facility and must have at least 12 air changes per hour (ACPH).

4. Final dosage forms of NIOSH Table 1 HDs and other HDs may be stored with non-HD drug inventory if permitted by entity policy in the Assessment of Risk.

G. Compounding with HDs
1. To help minimize the risk of exposure in a pharmacy compounding HDs, detailed standard operating procedures (SOPs) and training requirements must be developed. Workers must wear personal protective equipment (PPE) designed to be resistant to hazardous drugs. Goggles and face shields should be worn if splashing is possible, and respiratory protection should be worn if the HD is volatile or if particulate matter can become airborne.
2. Containment engineering controls to protect a preparation from microbial (if final preparation is to be sterile) and cross-contamination are required throughout the compounding procedures.
3. Containment engineering controls are divided into three types:
    a. Containment Primary Engineering Control (C-PEC);
    b. Containment Secondary Engineering Control (C-SEC); and
    c. Containment Supplemental Engineering Controls.
4. A C-PEC is a ventilated device designed to minimize the risk of exposure to the compounder and to the environment when HDs are handled directly. Containment Ventilated Enclosures (CVEs, often called powder containment hoods) are devices used only for nonsterile preparations. Biological Safety Cabinets (BSCs) and Compounding Aseptic Containment Isolators (CACIs) are used for sterile preparations and must maintain ISO 5 air cleanliness and have unidirectional airflow. The C-PEC must be operated continuously if used for sterile compounding or if it supplies some or all of the negative pressure for the room.

STUDY TIP: ISO class is determined by the number of particles larger than 0.5 microns in a volume of air. The smaller the ISO number, the cleaner the air. C-PECs must be ISO 5 or cleaner. Anterooms that open into a negative pressure room and buffer rooms must be ISO 7 or cleaner.

5. A C-SEC is the room in which the C-PEC is located. It can be a compounding suite (containing an anteroom and buffer room) or a containment segregated compounding area.

6. C-SECs must be used for compounding both nonsterile and sterile preparations and must:
   a. Be a room with fixed walls that is separate from non-hazardous storage or compounding;
   b. Have a negative pressure gradient of 0.010–0.030" of water column with respect to adjacent areas;
   c. Have appropriate air exchange (ACPH); and
   d. Be vented to the exterior of the facility.

STUDY TIP: The separate room and negative pressure work to contain the hazard. External ventilation and air changes per hour work to remove the hazard.

7. Containment supplemental engineering controls, such as closed system drug-transfer devices (CSTDs), provide additional protection from exposure of the compounder to one or more HDs. CSTDs must be used for administration of Table 1 NIOSH antineoplastics and should be used for compounding.
8. An eyewash station and other applicable emergency safety equipment (e.g., safety showers, fire blankets, etc.) meeting applicable laws and regulations must be readily available, and a sink must be available for hand washing. However, all water sources and drains must be located outside the buffer room and at least one meter from the C-PEC or entrance to any negative pressure room.
9. For entities where compounding of both sterile and nonsterile HDs is performed, the C-PECs must be located in separate rooms, unless the C-PECs used for nonsterile compounding can effectively maintain ISO 7 air quality in the room. If the C-PECs for nonsterile and sterile compounding are located in the same room, they must be placed at least one meter apart. If the C-PECs are in the same room, any nonsterile compounding that generates particulate matter may not be performed when sterile compounding is being performed.
10. A professional certifier must assess the primary and secondary engineering controls every six months. The C-PECs and C-SECs must meet the criteria listed in USP 797 (for facilities used for compounding sterile HDs) and USP 800 (for all facilities that compound HDs).

H. Nonsterile Compounding with HDs
   1. In addition to following the regulations set forth in this chapter, entities involved in compounding nonsterile preparation, regardless of whether the compounding involves HDs or not, must also comply with the requirements of USP Chapter 795, Pharmaceutical Compounding—Nonsterile Preparations.
   2. A C-PEC may not be required if the entity compounds only nonsterile, non-HD drugs, or if the entity is not manipulating HDs in any form except handling the final dosage forms (e.g., counting or repackaging tablets or capsules). This must be detailed in the Assessment of Risk.
   3. C-PECs used only for nonsterile HD compounding are negative pressure devices but are neither required to be ISO classified nor have unidirectional airflow.
   Requirements for C-PECs and C-SECs for compounding nonsterile HDs are summarized in the following table:

ENGINEERING CONTROLS FOR NONSTERILE HD COMPOUNDING

C-PEC	C-SEC
Externally vented (preferred) or redundant-HEPA filtered with HEPA filters in series	Room separate from nonhazardous activities
	Negative pressure (0.010–0.030-inch water column) relative to adjacent areas
	Externally vented
	12 ACPH

I. Sterile Compounding with HDs
   1. In addition to following the regulations set forth in this chapter, entities involved in compounding sterile preparation, regardless of whether the compounding involves HDs or not, must also comply with the requirements of USP Chapter 797, Pharmaceutical Compounding—Sterile Preparations.
   2. All C-PECs used for the purpose of compounding sterile hazardous drugs must be vented to the outside.
   3. As is the case with PECs used in the compounding of sterile non-HD preparations, C-PECs must maintain an ISO Class 5 or better air quality.
   4. Laminar airflow workbenches or Compounding Aseptic Isolators (CAIs) are not acceptable for compounding

antineoplastic HDs because they are positive pressure devices.

Requirements for C-PECs and C-SECs for compounding sterile HDs are summarized in the following table:

ENGINEERING CONTROLS FOR STERILE HD COMPOUNDING

C-SEC Configuration	C-PEC Requirements	C-SEC Requirements
ISO Class 7 buffers room with ISO Class 7 anteroom	• Vented Externally • Examples: Class II BSC or CACI	• Room separate from non-hazardous activities • Vented Externally • 30 ACPH • Positive pressure anteroom • Negative pressure as described previously in buffer room
Unclassified C-SCA	• Vented Externally • Examples: Class II BSC or CACI	• Room separate from non-hazardous activities • Vented Externally • 12 ACPH • Negative pressure as described previously

J. Documentation and Standard Operating Procedures (SOPs)
1. Any entity handling HDs must maintain SOPs for safe handling of HDs at all stages and locations where HDs are found in the facility.
2. These SOPs are to be reviewed at least annually and should include a hazard communication program, occupational safety program, designation of HD areas, and items discussed above.

K. Receiving, Labeling, Packaging, Transport, and Disposal
1. A facility must establish SOPs for the receiving, labeling, packaging, transport, and disposal of HDs.
2. Transport of HDs must be labeled, stored, and handled in accordance with applicable federal, state, and local regulations.
3. HDs must be transported in containers that minimize the risk of breakage and leakage.

L. Personnel Training
All personnel who handle HDs must be properly trained based on job function. The training must be documented.

M. Personal Protective Equipment
1. NIOSH documents provide guidance on personal protective equipment (PPE) such as not reusing disposable PPE and decontaminating reusable PPE.
2. Chapter 800 requires gowns, head and hair covers, shoe covers, and two pairs of powderless chemotherapy gloves when compounding either nonsterile or sterile antineoplastic agents. Two pairs of chemotherapy gloves and gowns resistant to permeability by HDs are also required when administering injectable antineoplastic HDs. One pair of chemo gloves must be worn when receiving NIOSH Table 1 antineoplastic HDs.
3. For other activities, the facility's SOPs must describe appropriate PPE to be worn. SOPs must be based on risk of exposure and activities.
4. At all stages of the handling of HDs, from receiving to waste disposal, PPE must be worn.
5. Chemotherapy gloves must meet the American Society of Testing Materials (ASTM) standard D6978 and should be worn when handling any HD. Chapter 800 states that chemotherapy gloves should be changed every 30 minutes unless the manufacturer recommends different intervals.
6. Chapter 800 states that gowns must close in the back, be disposable, and resist permeability of HDs. Gowns must be changed per the manufacturer's information for permeation of the gown. If there is no information from the manufacturer, then Chapter 800 states gowns are to be changed every 2–3 hours or immediately after a splash or spill. Personnel are not to wear in other areas of a facility the same gown that was worn in HD handling areas.
7. A second pair of shoe covers must be donned before entering the C-SEC and must be removed before leaving the HD handling areas and entering other areas of the facility.
8. Appropriate face and eye protection is to be worn when there is a risk of spills or splashes of HDs. Safety eyeglasses with side shields do not provide adequate protection.
9. When unpacking HDs not contained in plastic, personnel should wear elastomeric half-face masks which have been fit-tested with a P100 filter and a multi-gas cartridge.
10. All worn PPE should be considered contaminated and placed in an appropriate waste container to be disposed of properly.

PPE used in compounding HDs should be discarded in proper containers before leaving the C-SEC.
- **N.** Cleaning
  1. The cleaning process for hazardous drugs must start with deactivating the drug (when possible) and decontaminating the surfaces that the HDs have touched.
  2. After decontamination, the surfaces must be cleaned then disinfected.

STUDY TIP: Few HDs have specific information concerning how to deactivate them, so decontaminating the surfaces touched in the C-PEC and C-SEC is crucial. Decontamination is done with a properly diluted oxidizer or other agent intended to eliminate HDs. Cleaning is done with a properly diluted detergent. Disinfection is done with isopropyl alcohol, which must be sterile for use in C-PECs used for sterile compounding.

- **O.** Spill Control
  Facility policies must include the steps to take when a spill occurs.
- **P.** Medical Surveillance
  1. As part of a comprehensive exposure control program, medical surveillance complements all other attempts by Chapter 800 to minimize risks to healthcare workers. Medical surveillance is recommended but not required by USP 800.
  2. Elements of an appropriate medical surveillance program must be consistent with an entity's policies, and medical records should be consistent with regulations set forth by the Occupational Safety and Health Administration (OSHA).
  3. Chapter 800 outlines elements of a medical surveillance plan that should be included for all healthcare workers who may come into contact with hazardous drugs. The chapter also describes elements that should be included in a follow-up plan should HD exposure-related health changes occur. Again, the elements in the recommended medical surveillance and follow-up plans are not exhaustive, but they provide a good basis for the development of an appropriate program. Once again, however, any medical surveillance plan should follow entity policies.
- **Q.** Environmental Quality and Control
  1. While there are no currently accepted limits for HD surface contamination, Chapter 800 states that surface wipe

sampling for HDs should be performed routinely to ensure that cleaning procedures are effective in removing remaining HD residues after handling or compounding.
2. Surface wipe sampling should include, but not necessarily be limited to, the inside surface of the C-PEC and any equipment contained in it, pass-through chambers, staging surfaces, areas adjacent to the C-PEC, areas immediately outside the buffer room or C-SEC, and patient administration areas.
3. The chapter continues by saying that if any measurable HD residue is found, the designated person should consider taking actions such as reevaluating work practices, retraining personnel, etc.

IV. Florida Rules on Compounding
A. Compounding—Definition, Office Use Compounding, and Recordkeeping (Rules 64B16-27.700 and 64B16-28.140(4))
1. "Compounding" is the professional act by a pharmacist or other practitioner authorized by law, employing the science or art of any branch of the profession of pharmacy, incorporating ingredients to create a finished product for dispensing to a patient or for administration by a practitioner or practitioner's agent; and shall specifically include the professional act of preparing a unique finished product containing any ingredient or device defined by §§ 465.003(7) and (8). *Note: This is likely supposed to say §§ 465.003(8) "medicinal drugs" and (9) "patent or proprietary drugs (OTC)."*
Compounding includes:
   a. The preparation of drugs or devices in anticipation of prescriptions based on routine, regularly observed prescribing patterns;
   b. The preparation, pursuant to a prescription, of drugs or devices that are not commercially available;
   c. The preparation of commercially available products from bulk when the prescribing practitioner has prescribed the compounded product on a per-prescription basis, and the patient has been made aware that the compounded product will be prepared by the pharmacist. The reconstitution of commercially available products pursuant to the manufacturer's guidelines is permissible without notice to the practitioner.

2. The preparation of drugs or devices for sale or transfer to pharmacies or practitioners, or to entities for purposes of dispensing or distribution, is not compounding.

STUDY TIP: Compounding for practitioners to resale or distribute is not allowed, but compounding for administration in a practitioner's office is permitted. See "Office Use Compounding" below.

3. Office Use Compounding
   a. "Office Use" means the provision and administration of a compounded drug to a patient by a practitioner in the practitioner's office or in a healthcare facility or treatment setting, including a hospital, ambulatory surgical center, or pharmacy.
   b. A pharmacist may dispense and deliver a quantity of a compounded drug to a practitioner for office use, provided:
      (1) The quantity of a compounded drug does not exceed the amount a practitioner anticipated may be used in the practitioner's office before the expiration date of the drug;
      (2) The quantity of a compounded drug is reasonable considering the intended use of the compounded drug and the nature of the practitioner's practice;
      (3) The quantity of a compounded drug for any practitioner and all practitioners as a whole is not greater than the amount the pharmacy is capable of compounding in compliance with pharmaceutical standards for identity, strength, quality, and purity of the compounded drug that are consistent with USP guidelines and accreditation practices;
      (4) The pharmacy and the practitioner enter into a written agreement with specific provisions;
      (5) Adequate, retrievable records of all compounded drugs ordered by practitioners for office use are maintained as required by rule;
      (6) The label affixed to any compounded drug for office use includes:
         i. Name, address, and phone number of the compounding pharmacy;

ii. Name and strength of the preparation and list of active ingredients and strengths;
iii. Pharmacy's lot number and beyond-use date;
iv. Quantity or amount in the container;
v. Appropriate ancillary instructions such as storage instructions, cautionary statements, or hazardous drug warning labels where appropriate;
vi. The statement "For Institutional or Office Use Only—Not for Resale," or if provided to a veterinarian, the statement "Compounded Drug";
vii. For sterile products, the pharmacy must also be in compliance with requirements for outsourcing facilities. *See Chapter 1*

STUDY TIP: This rule allows office use compounding of nonsterile products that are not patient-specific. This may be in conflict with federal law, which only provides a mechanism for non-patient-specific sterile compounding through outsourcing (503B) facilities. Nevertheless, if a question on this appears on the MPJE, it is recommended to answer the question based on the Florida law.

4. Compounding Recordkeeping (Rule 64B16-28.140(4))
   A written record shall be maintained for each batch/sub-batch of a compounded product under the provisions of rule 64B16-27.700. This record shall include:
   a. Date of compounding;
   b. Control number for each batch/sub-batch of a compounded product:
      (1) This may be the manufacturer's lot number or new numbers assigned by the pharmacist.
      (2) If the number is assigned by the pharmacist, the pharmacist shall also record the original manufacturer's lot number and expiration dates.
      (3) If the original numbers and expiration dates are not known, the pharmacy shall record the source and acquisition date of the component.
   c. A complete formula for the compounded product maintained in a readily retrievable form, including methodology and necessary equipment;
   d. A signature or initials of the pharmacist or pharmacy technician performing the compounding;

e. A signature or initials of the pharmacist responsible for supervising pharmacy technicians involved in the compounding process;
   f. The name(s) of the manufacturer(s) of the raw materials used;
   g. The quantity in units of finished products or grams of raw materials;
   h. The package size and number of units prepared;
   i. The name of the patient who received the particular compounded product.
B. **Standards of Practice for Compounding Sterile Products (Rule 64B16-27.797)**
   Note: The provisions of Rule 64B16-27.797(5) on compounding that involves lyophilization of the sterile product have been moved to a separate section in this guide. See 4. below
   1. This rule adopts the standards of the following USP Chapters for all sterile product compounding in Florida with some variations or exceptions:
      a. Chapter 797—Pharmaceutical Compounding—Sterile Preparations
      b. Chapter 71—Sterility Tests
      c. Chapter 85—Bacterial Endotoxins Test
      d. Chapter 731—Loss on Drying
      Note: USP Chapters 71, 85, and 731 are not included in this book, but you should know that Florida has adopted those standards.

STUDY TIP: Florida has not adopted USP Chapter 795 on Compounding Nonsterile Preparations or USP Chapter 800 on Hazardous Drugs, but has adopted USP Chapter 797 (with some modifications). Since Florida has adopted USP 797, it is more likely that you would see questions on USP 797.

---

   2. Any pharmacy registered as an outsourcing facility must meet the current Good Manufacturing Practices (cGMPs) of FDA.
   3. Clarifications, variances, and exceptions:
      Note: These are areas where Florida has adopted rules different from USP 797, provided exceptions to certain requirements in USP 797, and added requirements not found in USP 797.
      a. Although USP requires the donning of gloves prior to entry into the clean-room, all required donning of gloves

can be performed after entry into the clean-room to avoid contamination of the gloves from the door handle or access device leading into the clean-room.

b. USP Chapter 797 requires that: "When closed-system vial-transfer devices (CSTDs) (i.e., vial-transfer systems that allow no venting or exposure of hazardous substance to the environment) are used, they shall be used within an ISO Class 5 environment of a BSC or CACI. The use of the CSTD is preferred because of their inherent closed-system process. In facilities that prepare a low volume of hazardous drugs, the use of two tiers of containment (e.g., CSTD within a BSC or CACI that is located in a non-negative pressure room) is acceptable." For the purpose of said provision, a "low volume of hazardous drugs" is defined as less than 40 doses per month.

c. USP Chapter 797 provides as follows in the "Facility Design and Environmental Controls" section: "An ISO Class 7 (see Table 1) buffer area and ante-area supplied with HEPA-filtered air shall receive an ACPH of not less than 30. The PEC is a good augmentation to generating air changes in the air supply of an area but cannot be the sole source of HEPA-filtered air. If the area has an ISO Class 5 (see Table 1) recirculating device, a minimum of 15 ACPHs through the area supplying HEPA filters is adequate, provided the combined ACPH is not less than 30. More air changes may be required, depending on the number of personnel and processes. HEPA-filtered supply air shall be introduced at the ceiling, and returns should be mounted low on the wall, creating a general top-down dilution of area air with HEPA-filtered make-up air. Ceiling-mounted returns are not recommended." Notwithstanding these provisions, pharmacies that meet the standards in this section as of the effective date of this rule are not required to change the location of supply air, return filters, or ducts, so long as the ISO standards are maintained.

d. USP Chapter 797 provides in part that the compounding facility's ceiling tiles located in the ante-area, buffer area, and clean-room that consist of inlaid panels "shall be impregnated with a polymer to render them impervious and hydrophobic, and they shall be caulked around each perimeter to seal them to the support frame." A pharmacy shall not be required to caulk the inlaid ceiling tiles to the perimeter of the support frame if the following conditions are met:

    (1) The ceiling tiles are specifically manufactured to be utilized in a facility that must meet and maintain an airborne particulate cleanliness of ISO Class 7 or better.

    (2) The core of the ceiling tiles are sealed on the front, back, and all edges to render them impervious and hydrophobic, so they can be properly maintained and cleaned as required by this rule.

    (3) The ceiling tiles are inlaid or installed using a gasket grid sealing system, which is manufactured for use in facilities that must meet and maintain an airborne particulate cleanliness of ISO Class 7 or better. The sealing system must create and maintain a positive seal between the ceiling tiles and the support frame, and the seal between the ceiling tiles and support frame shall be secured with retention clips.

4. Sterile compounded products prepared using a process that includes lyophilization shall, in addition to all applicable provisions of USP Chapter 797, be subject to the following additional requirements:

    a. Compounded sterile products prepared for lyophilization shall be maintained in ISO 5 unidirectional laminar flow air throughout sterilization, filling, and transport from the Primary Engineering Control ("PEC") into the lyophilizer. Smoke studies shall be conducted to demonstrate that transport from the PEC to the lyophilizer can be accomplished while maintaining ISO 5 laminar flow air at all times. The smoke study shall be recorded and available for inspection.

    b. The pharmacy shall establish, maintain, and follow policies and procedures for the high-level disinfection of the chamber, piping, and all other areas of the lyophilizer which pose a potential risk of contamination to the product.

    c. The pharmacy shall, initially and after any change to the cleaning process or agents, validate a high-level disinfection process for the lyophilizer. For the purposes of this rule, validation means that the high-level disinfection process shall be proven with validation studies performed with the 5 aerobic bacterial and fungal ATCC organisms referenced in USP Chapter 71. The validation studies must be performed by an external vendor or by an internal laboratory. A pharmacy with an internal laboratory shall be separated from the compounding area and the work area to prevent contamination in the pharmacy. Documentation of validation shall be readily available for inspection.

    d. A policy and procedure for cleaning the lyophilizer prior to high-level disinfection to include cleaning agents and schedules shall be established. Documentation of cleaning shall be maintained and readily available for inspection.

    e. The pharmacy shall establish policies and procedures as well as a schedule for the maintenance of the lyophilizer, which shall be, at a minimum, based on the manufacturer's recommendations. As leakage into the vacuum chamber poses a risk of contamination to the product, the maintenance schedule shall include provisions for periodically testing for leaks, along with all recommended procedures described by the equipment manufacturer. Documentation of routine maintenance shall be available for inspection.

    f. The pharmacy shall develop standard operating procedures (SOPs) and a quality assurance program to include validation of the filling process, container closure integrity, the frequent monitoring of fill volumes, training and assessment of personnel involved in all aspects of compounding sterile products for lyophilization, identification of overfills and underfills, equipment qualification, formula verification, and evaluation of the finished product for conformance to specifications.

    g. The pharmacy shall establish provisions for sterilizing the inert gas or air used for backfilling during the vacuum release phase. Filters shall be used to sterilize the gas or air and shall undergo the manufacturer's recommended integrity testing.

    h. Media fills shall be conducted using maximum batch sizes. The media fills shall demonstrate the filling, transportation to the lyophilizer, loading, and stoppering operations. Media shall not be frozen as part of the media fill as freezing of the media could reduce the ability of the media to support growth.

i. Personnel preparing sterile compounds for lyophilization shall wear sterile Personal Protective Equipment (PPE) that allows all exposed skin to be covered.

j. Personnel shall perform Glove Fingertip Sampling with each batch after the fill and transport of the vials. This sampling shall be documented and incorporated into the batch record.

k. In-process acceptance criteria for each lyophilized product shall be established and may include criteria such as color, moisture limits, and visual appearance. A 100% visual examination of the finished product shall be conducted to determine that the product conforms to the established visual criteria. This examination shall be documented and incorporated in the batch record.

l. Laboratory testing.

  (1) Finished product testing shall be conducted on all batches. Procedures for selecting samples from the batch for testing shall be written and followed. Procedures may include location of vials in the lyophilizer (e.g., select from each corner and the middle of each shelf) and position in the fill line (e.g., beginning, middle, and end of fill).

  (2) Finished product testing for all batches shall include sterility testing with methods described in USP Chapter 71, unless an alternative method has been validated and shown to be equivalent or better. Diluents for reconstituting the vials for testing shall be preservative free. Lyophilized products released with beyond-use dates within USP Chapter 797 guidelines shall, in lieu of sterility testing, conduct viable air, surface, and personnel (gloves and sleeves) sampling for each batch.

  (3) Endotoxin limits shall be established for every lyophilized product.

  (4) Endotoxin testing for all lyophilized batches shall be performed in accordance with USP Chapter 85 and

confirmed to fall within the set limits. This shall be documented on the batch record.

(5) Potency, radiochemical purity, or applicable tests to assure label claim shall be conducted on every batch and documented in the batch record. In lieu of potency testing, weight-based verification may occur based on formula verification. Weight-based verification will be based on 90%–110% theoretical yield. Potency testing shall be based on USP monograph if one is available; if not, it shall be based on 90%–110% theoretical yield.

(6) Initial potency testing shall be established based on worst-case scenario.

CHAPTER SIX
Disciplinary Actions and Procedures, and Miscellaneous Laws and Rules

CHAPTER SIX
Disciplinary Actions and Procedures, and Miscellaneous Laws and Rules

I. **Disciplinary Actions and Procedures**
   A. Authority to Inspect (§ 465.017)
      1. Duly authorized agents and employees of the department may inspect in a lawful manner at all reasonable hours any pharmacy, hospital, clinic, wholesale establishment, manufacturer, physician's office, or any other place in the state in which drugs and medical supplies are compounded, manufactured, packed, packaged, made, stored, sold, offered for sale, exposed for sale, or kept for sale for the purpose of:
         a. Determining if any provision of this chapter or any rule adopted under its authority is being violated;
         b. Securing samples or specimens of any drug or medical supply after paying or offering to pay for such sample or specimen; or
         c. Securing such other evidence as may be needed for prosecution under this chapter.
      2. Duly authorized agents and employees of the department may inspect a registered nonresident pharmacy or a registered nonresident sterile compounding permittee. The costs of such inspections shall be borne by such pharmacy or permittee.
   B. Grounds for Denial of a License or Disciplinary Action (§ 465.016)
   Note: The grounds of discipline listed below are from the Pharmacy Act, but pharmacists are also subject to some of the grounds for discipline applicable to all healthcare practitioners under the Florida Department of Health. See Florida statute § 456.072.
      1. Obtaining license by misrepresentation or fraud or through an error of the Board or Department.
      2. Procuring or attempting to procure a license for another person.
      3. Permitting person not licensed as a pharmacist in this state or not registered as an intern in this state, or permitting a registered intern who is not acting under the direct and immediate supervision of a licensed pharmacist to fill,

compound, or dispense any prescription in a pharmacy owned or operated by such pharmacist or in a pharmacy where such pharmacist is employed or on duty.

4. Being unfit or incompetent to practice pharmacy by reason of:
   a. Habitual intoxication;
   b. Misuse or abuse of any controlled substance; or
   c. Abnormal physical or mental condition which threatens the public safety.
5. Violating the federal Food, Drug and Cosmetic Act or federal Controlled Substances Act.
6. Having been convicted or found guilty, regardless of adjudication, of a crime which directly relates to the ability to practice pharmacy. A plea of nolo contendere (no contest) constitutes a conviction for purposes of this section.
7. Using, in the compounding or dispensing of a prescription, an ingredient or article different in any matter from the ingredient or article prescribed (except as authorized for generic substitution or a formulary system).
8. Having been disciplined by a regulatory authority in another state for any offense that would be a violation of the pharmacy act.
9. Compounding, dispensing, or distributing legend drugs or controlled substances other than in the course of the professional practice of pharmacy.
10. Making or filing a report or record known to be false, intentionally or negligently failing to file a report or record required by state or federal law, or willfully impeding or obstructing such filing or inducing another person to do so.
11. Failing to make prescription fee or price information readily available upon request.
12. Placing in the stock of any pharmacy any part of a prescription that has been returned by a patient (exception for unit-dose medication in hospitals, nursing homes, etc.).
13. Being unable to practice pharmacy with reasonable skill and safety by reason of illness, use of drugs, narcotics, chemicals, or any other type of material or as a result of any mental or physical condition.

STUDY TIP: Despite these provisions, many cases of impairment due to alcohol, drugs, or mental or physical issues do not result in discipline. Florida has an impaired practitioner program called the Professionals Resource Network (PRN). A pharmacist with an impairment who voluntarily enters into a contract for treatment with PRN will not be referred to the Board for discipline as long as they acknowledge the impairment and successfully complete the program. The Board may also refer pharmacists to the PRN program if they receive a complaint regarding impairment under certain circumstances. For more information, see *www.flprn.org*

14. Violating a rule of the Board or Department or violating an order previously entered in a disciplinary hearing.
15. Failing to report to the Department a physician who the pharmacist knows has violated the grounds for disciplinary action set out in the law under which that person is licensed and who provides healthcare services in a facility licensed under Chapter 395 (hospitals and other licensed facilities) or an HMO in which the pharmacist also provides service. However, a person who the licensee knows is unable to practice medicine or osteopathic medicine with reasonable skill and safety to patients by reason of illness or use of alcohol, drugs, narcotics, chemicals, or any other type of material, or as a result of a mental or physical condition, may be reported to a consultant operating an impaired practitioner (PRN) program rather than to the Department.

STUDY TIP: While this rule only discusses reporting of impaired physicians that work in the same facilities as a pharmacist, it is recommended that a pharmacist refer any impaired co-worker to the Florida Professionals Recovery Network (PRN).

16. Failing to notify the Board in writing within 20 days of the commencement or cessation of practice when such commencement or cessation of practice was a result of a pending or completed disciplinary action or investigation in another jurisdiction.
17. Using or releasing a patient's records except as authorized.
18. Violating any provision of Chapter 456 or 465 and any rules adopted pursuant thereto.
19. Dispensing any medicinal drug based upon a communication that purports to be a prescription when the pharmacist knows or has reason to believe that the purported

prescription is not based upon a valid practitioner-patient relationship.
20. Committing an error or omission during the performance of a specific function of prescription drug processing, which includes, for purposes of this paragraph:
   a. Receiving, interpreting, or clarifying a prescription.
   b. Entering prescription data into the pharmacy's record.
   c. Verifying or validating a prescription.
   d. Performing pharmaceutical calculations.
   e. Performing prospective drug review as defined by the Board.
   f. Obtaining refill and substitution authorizations.
   g. Interpreting or acting on clinical data.
   h. Performing therapeutic interventions.
   i. Providing drug information concerning a patient's prescription.
   j. Providing patient counseling.

C. Other Violations (§ 465.015)

Note: Some of these violations are criminal violations and are applicable to any person (not just pharmacists or pharmacy technicians) while other ones are specific to pharmacists or pharmacy technicians.

1. It is unlawful for any person to own, operate, maintain, open, establish, conduct, or have charge of, either alone or with another person or persons, a pharmacy:
   a. Which is not registered under the provisions of this chapter.
   b. In which a person not licensed as a pharmacist in this state or not registered as an intern in this state, or in which an intern who is not acting under the direct and immediate personal supervision of a licensed pharmacist fills, compounds, or dispenses any prescription or dispenses medicinal drugs.
2. It is unlawful for any person:
   a. To make a false or fraudulent statement, either for herself or himself or for another person, in any application, affidavit, or statement presented to the Board or in any proceeding before the Board.
   b. To fill, compound, or dispense prescriptions or to dispense medicinal drugs if such person does not hold an active license as a pharmacist in this state, is not

registered as an intern in this state, or is an intern not acting under the direct and immediate personal supervision of a licensed pharmacist.
- c. To sell or dispense medicinal drugs without first being furnished with a prescription.
- d. To sell samples or complimentary packages of drug products.
3. It is unlawful for any person other than a pharmacist licensed under this chapter to use the title "pharmacist" or "druggist" or otherwise lead the public to believe that she or he is engaged in the practice of pharmacy.
4. It is unlawful for any person other than an owner of a pharmacy registered under this chapter to display any sign or to take any other action that would lead the public to believe that such person is engaged in the business of compounding, dispensing, or retailing any medicinal drugs. This paragraph shall not preclude a person not licensed as a pharmacist from owning a pharmacy.
5. It is unlawful for a person, firm, or corporation that is not licensed or registered under this chapter to:
   - a. Use in a trade name, sign, letter, or advertisement any term, including "drug," "pharmacy," "prescription drugs," "Rx," or "apothecary," which implies that the person, firm, or corporation is licensed or registered to practice pharmacy in this state.
   - b. Hold himself or herself out to others as a person, firm, or corporation licensed or registered to practice pharmacy in this state.
6. It is unlawful for a person who is not registered as a pharmacy technician under this chapter, or who is not otherwise exempt from the requirement to register as a pharmacy technician, to perform the functions of a registered pharmacy technician, or hold himself or herself out to others as a person who is registered to perform the functions of a registered pharmacy technician in this state.

D. Board Action on Pharmacy Permit Applicants (§ 465.022(5) and (6))
1. The Department or Board *shall* deny an application for a pharmacy permit if the applicant or an affiliated person, partner, officer, director, or prescription department manager or consultant pharmacist of record of the applicant:

a. Has obtained a permit by misrepresentation or fraud.
b. Has attempted to procure, or has procured, a permit for any other person by making, or causing to be made, any false representation.
c. Has been convicted of, or entered a plea of guilty or nolo contendere to, regardless of adjudication, a crime in any jurisdiction which relates to the practice of, or the ability to practice, the profession of pharmacy.
d. Has been convicted of, or entered a plea of guilty or nolo contendere to, regardless of adjudication, a crime in any jurisdiction which relates to healthcare fraud.
e. Has been convicted of, or entered a plea of guilty or nolo contendere to, regardless of adjudication, a felony under Chapter 409, Chapter 817, or Chapter 893, or a similar felony offense committed in another state or jurisdiction, since July 1, 2009.
f. Has been convicted of, or entered a plea of guilty or nolo contendere to, regardless of adjudication, a felony under 21 U.S.C. ss. 801–970 or 42 U.S.C. ss. 1395–1396 since July 1, 2009.
g. Has been terminated for cause from the Florida Medicaid program unless the applicant has been in good standing with the Florida Medicaid program for the most recent 5-year period.
h. Has been terminated for cause, pursuant to the appeals procedures established by the state, from any other state Medicaid program, unless the applicant has been in good standing with a state Medicaid program for the most recent 5-year period and the termination occurred at least 20 years before the date of the application.
i. Is currently listed on the United States Department of Health and Human Services Office of Inspector General's List of Excluded Individuals and Entities.
j. Has dispensed any medicinal drug based upon a communication that purports to be a prescription as defined when the pharmacist knows or has reason to believe that the purported prescription is not based upon a valid practitioner-patient relationship that includes a documented patient evaluation, including history and a physical examination adequate to establish the diagnosis for which any drug is prescribed and any other requirement

established by Board rule under Chapter 458, Chapter 459, Chapter 461, Chapter 463, Chapter 464, or Chapter 466.
2. The Department or Board may deny an application for a pharmacy permit if the applicant or an affiliated person, partner, officer, director, or prescription department manager or consultant pharmacist of record of the applicant has violated or failed to comply with any provision of this chapter; Chapter 499, the Florida Drug and Cosmetic Act; Chapter 893; 21 U.S.C. ss. 301–392, the Federal Food, Drug, and Cosmetic Act; 21 U.S.C. ss. 821 et seq., the Comprehensive Drug Abuse Prevention and Control Act; or any rules or regulations promulgated thereunder unless the violation or noncompliance is technical.

E. Disciplinary Action (§ 465.023)
1. The Department or the Board may revoke or suspend the permit of any pharmacy permittee, and may fine, place on probation, or otherwise discipline any pharmacy permittee if the permittee, or any affiliated person, partner, officer, director, or agent of the permittee, including a person fingerprinted under § 465.022(3), has:
   a. Obtained a permit by misrepresentation or fraud or through an error of the Department or the Board;
   b. Attempted to procure, or has procured, a permit for any other person by making, or causing to be made, any false representation;
   c. Violated any of the requirements of this chapter (465) or any of the rules of the Board of Pharmacy; of Chapter 499, known as the "Florida Drug and Cosmetic Act"; of 21 U.S.C. ss. 301–392, known as the "Federal Food, Drug, and Cosmetic Act"; of 21 U.S.C. ss. 821 et seq., known as the "Comprehensive Drug Abuse Prevention and Control Act"; or of Chapter 893;
   d. Been convicted or found guilty, regardless of adjudication, of a felony or any other crime involving moral turpitude in any of the courts of this state, of any other state, or of the United States;
   e. Been convicted or disciplined by a regulatory agency of the Federal Government or a regulatory agency of another state for any offense that would constitute a violation of this chapter;

- f. Been convicted of, or entered a plea of guilty or nolo contendere to, regardless of adjudication, a crime in any jurisdiction which relates to the practice of, or the ability to practice, the profession of pharmacy; *Note: All healthcare licensees, including pharmacists, must report to their respective Board any conviction or pleas of nolo contendere to any crime in writing within 30 days. See § 456.072(1)(x)*
- g. Been convicted of, or entered a plea of guilty or nolo contendere to, regardless of adjudication, a crime in any jurisdiction which relates to healthcare fraud; or
- h. Dispensed any medicinal drug based upon a communication that purports to be a prescription when the pharmacist knows or has reason to believe that the purported prescription is not based upon a valid practitioner-patient relationship that includes a documented patient evaluation, including history and a physical examination adequate to establish the diagnosis for which any drug is prescribed and any other requirement established by Board rule under Chapter 458, Chapter 459, Chapter 461, Chapter 463, Chapter 464, or Chapter 466.

2. If a pharmacy permit is revoked or suspended, the owner, manager, or proprietor shall cease to operate the establishment as a pharmacy as of the effective date of such suspension or revocation.
    - a. In the event of such revocation or suspension, the owner, manager, or proprietor shall remove from the premises all signs and symbols identifying the premises as a pharmacy.
    - b. The period of such suspension shall be prescribed by the Board of Pharmacy, but in no case shall it exceed 1 year.
    - c. In the event that the permit is revoked, the person owning or operating the establishment shall not be entitled to make application for a permit to operate a pharmacy for a period of 1 year from the date of such revocation.
    - d. Upon the effective date of such revocation, the permittee shall advise the Board of Pharmacy of the disposition of the medicinal drugs located on the premises. Such disposition shall be subject to continuing supervision and approval by the Board of Pharmacy.

F. Disciplinary Guidelines (Rule 64B16-30.001)
   1. This rule sets out a comprehensive list of the range of disciplinary penalties that will be imposed upon a licensee that is found guilty of specific violations.
   2. The Board can deviate from the guidelines upon a showing of aggravating or mitigating circumstances by clear and convincing evidence.
   3. Aggravating circumstances serve to increase the penalty imposed and include:
      a. History of previous violations of the practice act and rules;
      b. In the case of negligent acts, the magnitude and scope of damage or potential damage inflicted upon the patient or the public;
      c. Evidence of violation of professional practice acts in other jurisdictions where the licensee has been disciplined by the appropriate regulatory authority; and
      d. Harm that occurred.
   4. Mitigating circumstances serve to decrease the penalty imposed and include:
      a. In the case of negligent acts, the minor nature of the damage or potential damage to the patient or the public;
      b. Lack of previous disciplinary history in Florida or any other jurisdiction;
      c. Restitution of any monetary damage suffered by the patient;
      d. The licensee's professional standing among his or her peers;
      e. Steps already taken by the licensee to ensure the non-occurrence of similar violations in the future; and
      f. The degree of financial hardship incurred by the imposition of fines or suspension.
   5. All fines imposed by the Board must be paid within 90 days from the date of the final order unless that time limitation has been modified by the Board for good cause in order to prevent undue hardship.
G. Minor Violations (Rule 64B16-30.002 and Florida Statute § 456.073(3))
   1. Florida law requires each Board under the Department of Health to establish, by rule, a list of violations that are considered minor violations for an initial offence. For these

minor violations which do not endanger the public health, safety, and welfare and which do not demonstrate a serious inability to practice the profession, the Board may issue a Notice of Noncompliance.

Note: The Board of Pharmacy rule calls them Notice of Deficiencies.

2. Minor Violations include:
   a. Outdated pharmaceuticals (Rule 64B16-28.110);
   b. Failure to meet regulation of daily operating hours (Rule 64B16-28.404);
   c. Generic substitution sign not displayed (§ 465.025(7));
   d. Information required on controlled substance prescriptions: practitioner's address, practitioner's DEA registration number, patient's address (FLCSA § 893.04);
   e. Failure by dispensing pharmacists to have certified the daily hard-copy printout or daily log (Rule 64B16-28.140(3)(c) or (e));
   f. Failure to have pharmacy minimally equipped, i.e., references, compounding equipment, and a current copy of the laws and rules governing the practice of pharmacy in the State of Florida (Rule 64B16-28.107);
   g. Failure to properly identify pharmacy technicians (Rule 64B16-27.410);
   h. Results of P&E quality assurance program not documented or available for inspection (Rule 64B16-28.820(3)(d));
   i. Improper storage of legend drugs (Rule 64B16-28.120);
   j. Improper documentation of destruction of controlled substances (Rules 64B16-28.301 and 64B16-28.303);
   k. Consultant pharmacist's monthly reports not current or available for inspection (Rules 64B16-28.501 and 64B16-28.702(2));
   l. Controlled substance prescription labels lack transfer crime warning labeling (Rule 64B16-28.502(2)(c));
   m. Failure to maintain proof of licensure, display licenses/registrations or notices, or to properly identify pharmacy staff (Rule 64B16-27.100); and
   n. Failure to have a continuously designated Prescription Department Manager or Consultant Pharmacist of Record, if the gap between designations is less than 15 business days (Rules 64B16-27.450 and 64B16-28.501).

3. The Department's investigator may issue a Notice of Deficiencies when the above conditions occur. In such cases, licensees shall correct the violation and respond to the investigator on forms provided by the Department and with other evidence of compliance as may be necessary, within 30 days, to certify current compliance. Failure to do so shall subject the licensee to further proceedings.
4. A Notice of Deficiencies is not considered disciplinary action.

H. Citations (Florida Statute § 456.077 and Rule 64B16-30.003)
1. Florida law requires each Board under the Department of Health to establish, by rule, a list of violations for which a citation may be issued. Citation violations are those violations for which there is no substantial threat to the public health, safety, and welfare or no violation of standard of care involving injury to a patient. A citation may include a penalty (fine) and payment of the costs of investigation.
2. A citation is not considered disciplinary action for the first offense.
3. Citation violations include:
   a. Practicing pharmacy as an inactive licensee;
   b. Operating a pharmacy with an inactive permit;
   c. First-time failure to complete the required continuing education requirements during the biennial license period;
   d. Failure to timely pay a fine or costs incurred by a Board order;
   e. Failure to display any sign, license, or permit required by statute or rule;
   f. Failure to have any reference material required by statute or rule available;
   g. Failure to notify the Board of a change in prescription department manager or consultant pharmacist;
   h. Using, in the compounding of a prescription, or furnishing upon a prescription, any ingredient or article different in any manner from the ingredient or article prescribed or dispensing a medication with dosage form instructions different in any way than prescribed, provided that the medication was not used or ingested;
   i. Tendering a check payable to the Board of Pharmacy or Department of Health that is dishonored;

- j. Failure to comply with the educational course requirements for HIV/AIDS;
- k. Failure to correct minor violations;
- l. First-time failure to report controlled substance dispensing information to the PDMP;
- m. First-time failure to consult the PDMP prior to dispensing a controlled substance;
- n. Failure to request a photo or other verification of identity prior to dispensing a controlled substance to a person not known;
- o. Failure to inform customers of a less expensive drug when cost-sharing obligation to customer exceeds retail price;
- p. Failure to comply with pharmacist to registered pharmacy technician ratio for activities not involving sterile compounding with no injury to patient; and
- q. Failure to remove from active stock and properly quarantine outdated prescription drugs.

I. Overview of Disciplinary Procedure
1. Complaints against pharmacies, pharmacists, registered pharmacy technicians, and registered pharmacy interns made to the Board of Pharmacy are investigated by the Medical Quality Assurance Division of the Florida Department of Health.
2. If the complaint is not considered a minor violation or one that can be resolved with a citation, formal disciplinary action may be taken.
3. The Department will notify the subject of the complaint and provide the subject an opportunity to submit a response. After a thorough investigation, the complaint is forwarded to the prosecution services unit where an attorney reviews the file and recommends either dismissal or the filing of an administrative complaint.
4. The Department then makes a final recommendation to a Probable Cause Panel on the complaint within six months of its receipt.
5. The Probable Cause Panel is composed of at least two Board members. The Probable Cause Panel is given a copy of the Department's complete investigative file, any expert opinions obtained by the Department, and the subject's response to the complaint, if one was submitted.

6. The Probable Cause Panel determines whether a complaint should be closed or an administrative complaint filed. A decision to either find probable cause on a complaint or to dismiss it must be made by a majority vote of the Probable Cause Panel.
7. If probable cause is found, a complaint is filed and the subject has 21 days to respond.
8. The subject of a complaint may request a formal administrative hearing before an Administrative Law Judge or an informal hearing before the Board. Regardless of the type of hearing requested, a complaint can also be settled through a consent decree or stipulation which is submitted to the Board for approval.
9. Any Board member who participated on the Probable Cause Panel for a complaint may not vote on the final disciplinary decision for that complaint.

II. Miscellaneous Laws and Rules
   A. Administration of Antipsychotic Medication by Injection (§ 465.1893)
   1. A pharmacist, at the direction of a licensed physician, may administer a long-acting antipsychotic medication approved by the FDA by injection to a patient if the pharmacist:
      a. Is authorized by and acting within the framework of an established protocol with the prescribing physician.
      b. Practices at a facility that accommodates privacy for non-deltoid injections and conforms with state rules and regulations regarding the appropriate and safe disposal of medication and medical waste.
      c. Has completed the course required below.
   2. A separate prescription from a physician is required for each injection administered by a pharmacist.
   3. A pharmacist seeking to administer a long-acting antipsychotic medication by injection must complete an 8-hour continuing education course that concerns the safe and effective administration of behavioral health and antipsychotic medications by injection, including, but not limited to, potential allergic reactions to such medications. The course can count toward the required 30 hours of pharmacist continuing education for license renewal.

B. Dispensing Practitioner (§ 465.0276)
1. A practitioner authorized by law to prescribe drugs may dispense such drugs to her or his patients in the regular course of her or his practice in compliance with this section.
2. A practitioner who dispenses medicinal drugs for human consumption for a fee or remuneration of any kind, whether direct or indirect, must:
   a. Register with her or his professional licensing board as a dispensing practitioner and pay a fee at the time of such registration and upon each renewal of her or his license.
   b. Comply with and be subject to all laws and rules applicable to pharmacists and pharmacies.
   c. Before dispensing any drug, give the patient a written prescription and orally or in writing advise the patient that the prescription may be filled in the practitioner's office or at any pharmacy.
3. A dispensing practitioner may not dispense a controlled substance listed in Schedule II or Schedule III. This restriction does not apply to:
   a. The dispensing of complimentary packages of medicinal drugs which are labeled as a drug sample or complimentary drug to a practitioner's own patients in the regular course of her or his practice without the payment of a fee or remuneration of any kind, whether direct or indirect.
   b. The dispensing of controlled substances in the healthcare system of the Department of Corrections.
   c. The dispensing of a controlled substance listed in Schedule II or Schedule III in connection with the performance of a surgical procedure under the following conditions:
      (1) For a Schedule II opioid drug for the treatment of acute pain, the 3- or 7-day supply limits apply. *See Chapter 2, Section IX*
      (2) For the treatment of pain other than acute pain, a practitioner must indicate "NONACUTE PAIN" on a prescription.
      (3) For the treatment of pain related to a traumatic injury with an Injury Severity Score of 9 or greater, a practitioner must concurrently prescribe an emergency opioid antagonist.
      (4) For a controlled substance listed in Schedule III, the amount dispensed may not exceed a 14-day supply.

d. The dispensing of a controlled substance listed in Schedule II or Schedule III pursuant to an approved clinical trial.
   e. The dispensing of methadone in a facility licensed under § 397.427 where medication-assisted treatment for opiate addiction is provided.
   f. The dispensing of a controlled substance listed in Schedule II or Schedule III to a patient of a hospice facility.
   g. The dispensing of controlled substances listed in Schedule II or Schedule III which have been approved by the United States Food and Drug Administration for the purpose of treating opiate addictions, including, but not limited to, buprenorphine and buprenorphine combination products, by an authorized practitioner authorized to the practitioner's own patients for the medication-assisted treatment of opiate addiction.
4. A practitioner who confines her or his activities to the dispensing of complimentary packages of medicinal drugs to the practitioner's own patients in the regular course of her or his practice, without the payment of a fee or remuneration of any kind, whether direct or indirect, and who herself or himself dispenses such drugs is not required to register as a dispensing practitioner. The practitioner must dispense such drugs in the manufacturer's labeled package with the practitioner's name, patient's name, and date dispensed, or, if such drugs are not dispensed in the manufacturer's labeled package, they must be dispensed in a container which bears the following information:
   a. Practitioner's name;
   b. Patient's name;
   c. Date dispensed;
   d. Name and strength of drug; and
   e. Directions for use.
5. This law does not prohibit a licensed veterinarian from administering a compounded drug to a patient or dispensing a compounded drug to the patient's owner or caretaker.
C. Sale of Syringes and Needles
   1. Florida law does not require a prescription to sell syringes or needles to a person 18 years of age or over.
   2. A prescription is required for persons under 18 years of age.

D. Standards of Practice for Orthotics and Pedorthics (§ 465.1901 and Rule 64B16-27.850)
1. Although the Florida Department of Health licenses practitioners of orthotics and pedorthics under FS 468.803, the FPA specifically exempts pharmacists from those provisions.
2. This means that a pharmacist may, pursuant to written prescription, participate in the evaluation treatment formulation, measuring, designing, fabricating, assembling, fitting, adjusting, servicing, or providing initial training to accomplish the fitting of an orthosis or pedorthic device.
3. If a patient is under the care of a licensed occupational therapist or physical therapist, the pharmacist must consult with the therapist if the therapist has requested consultation.
4. The pharmacist's professional responsibilities include:
   a. Ongoing consultation with the prescribing physician.
   b. Orthotic and/or pedorthic evaluation of the patient.
   c. Identification and documentation of precautions, special problems, or contraindications.
   d. Development, implementation of, and periodic review of a treatment plan.
   e. Collaboration with other members of the healthcare team.
   f. Advising the patient of the nature of the purpose and nature of the services to be rendered and the techniques for use and care of the devices.
   g. Determination of the appropriateness of proper fit and function of the devices.
5. The Infectious Disease Elimination Act (IDEA) was passed into law in Florida in 2019 and allows counties to set up needle and syringe exchange programs.

CHAPTER SEVEN
Summary Charts and Self-Assessment Questions

SUMMARY CHART OF DAYS' SUPPLY LIMITATIONS

This chart summarizes various laws and rules that limit the days' supply that may be prescribed or dispensed.

Applicable To	Days' Supply Limit	Reference
Drugs dispensed by practitioner from an Emergency Room	24-hour supply or minimal dispensing quantity	Rule 64B16-28.6021
Emergency Verbal Schedule II Prescription	72-hour supply	FLCSA § 893.04(1)(f)
Emergency Refill (not Governor-declared emergency)	72-hour supply	FPA § 464.0275
Prescriptions for Schedule II Opioids for Acute Pain	3-day supply	Florida Statute 456.44
Drugs dispensed by a hospital under a Special—Limited Community Pharmacy Permit	3-day supply	Rule 64B16-28.810
Unable to check PDMP because system is down or technological failure.	3-day supply	FLCSA § 893.055(8)(b)
Prescriptions from Certified Optometrists for oral analgesics and anti-glaucoma agent on approved formulary	3-day supply—unless optometrist consults with a licensed physician	Florida Statute 463.0055(3)
Schedule II prescription from APRNs* *Exception for psychiatric nurses	7-day supply* *Additional restrictions for opioids for acute pain	Florida Statute 464.012(6)(a) and Rule 64B9-4.016
Schedule II prescriptions from Physician Assistants	7-day supply* *Additional requirements for opioids for acute pain	Florida Statute 458.347(4)(f)(1) and Rule 64B8-30.008
Prescription for Opioid for Acute Pain with "Acute Pain Exception" on the Prescription	7-day supply	Florida Statute 465.44
Dispensing of a Schedule III drug by a dispensing practitioner	14-day supply	FPA § 465.0276
Verbal Schedule III prescription	30-day supply	FLCSA § 893.05(2)(e)
Emergency Refill—Governor-declared emergency	30-day supply	FPA § 464.0275
Pharmacist Order for Medicinal Drugs	34-day supply	FPA § 464.186
Multiple Schedule II prescriptions issued on the same day	90-day supply	21 CFR 14016.12(b)(1)

SUMMARY CHART OF NOTIFICATION, REPORTING, AND OTHER TIME-LIMITED REQUIREMENTS

This chart summarizes the major laws and rules that have a specific time limit or time frame for notification, reporting, or specific actions.

Notification or Action Required	Notification or Reporting to	Time Limit
Notification of illegitimate product	Trading partners	24 hours
Theft or significant loss of controlled substances	DEA County Sheriff and Board of Pharmacy	Within one business day 24 hours
Person obtaining or attempting to obtain controlled substances fraudulently	County Sheriff or other chief law enforcement agency of county	24 hours
Reporting of controlled substances dispensed	PDMP	Close of next business day after dispensing
Completed and witnessed DEA Form 41 for Destruction of Drugs	DEA (but Florida requirement)	Within one business day of destruction
Notification of commencement of operations for a community pharmacy	Board of Pharmacy	Within 2 days of commencement of operations
Print out a hard-copy record from computer of all prescriptions dispensed	N/A	Within 48 hours of request
Print out a hard-copy record from computer of a summary record of controlled substance prescriptions dispensed	N/A	Within 72 hours of request
Time limit to dispense remaining quantity of a partially filled Schedule II prescription if the pharmacist is unable to supply full quantity	N/A	72 hours
Print out the daily hard-copy record from computer of all prescriptions dispensed	N/A	72 hours* *Note—most pharmacies do not do this and use logbook instead
Administration of narcotics to an addicted individual by a practitioner or hospital	N/A	3 days

Notification or Action Required	Notification or Reporting to	Time Limit
Time to obtain written or electronic prescription from practitioner after dispensing an emergency verbal Schedule II prescription	N/A	7 days
Required backup of pharmacy computer system	N/A	Weekly
Pharmacist signing of daily hard-copy printout of prescriptions dispensed	N/A	7 days
Change in Prescription Department Manager	Board of Pharmacy	10 days
Change in Consultant Pharmacist of Record	Board of Pharmacy	10 days
Election to delay commencement of operations in a community pharmacy	Board of Pharmacy	14 days
Notification of commencement or cessation of practice as a result of pending or completed disciplinary action in another jurisdiction	Board of Pharmacy	20 days
Time to respond to a complaint	Board of Pharmacy	21 days
Time limit to dispense remaining quantity of a partially filled Schedule II prescription if the patient or prescriber makes the request	N/A	30 days
Termination of enrollment in intern program or registration or attendance at college or school of pharmacy	Board of Pharmacy	30 days
Time limit to dispense remaining quantity of a partially filled Schedule II prescription if it is for an LTCF or hospice patient	N/A	60 days
Notification of breach of unsecured Protected Health Information (PHI)	Affected individual	60 calendar days
Payment of fines	Department of Health	90 days
Written notice of reason for failure to commence operations of a community pharmacy	Board of Pharmacy	6 months
Suspension of license	N/A	Not to exceed 1 year
Reapplication after revocation	N/A	At least 1 year

SELF-ASSESSMENT QUESTIONS

The following questions are designed to test your knowledge of the material in this book. The author has no knowledge of specific questions on the Florida MPJE and has developed these questions independently. No representation is made that these questions are similar to actual questions on the MPJE. An answer key with explanations follows at the end of this section.

1. In order to enter into a collaborative practice agreement with a physician for patients with a chronic health condition, a pharmacist must complete an initial course of
   a. 8 hours
   b. 15 hours
   c. 20 hours
   d. 30 hours

2. A pharmacist who is certified to test and treat for minor, non-chronic health conditions may test and treat which of the following? **Select all that apply.**
   a. Diabetes
   b. Streptococcus
   c. Lice
   d. Asthma

3. You receive a prescription calling for you to compound and dispense a 1-pint bottle of a solution containing 120 mg of acetaminophen and 16 mg of codeine per teaspoon with cherry flavoring. What schedule would this product be in?
   a. Schedule II
   b. Schedule III
   c. Schedule IV
   d. Schedule V

4. DEA registrations beginning with the letter M are issued to
   a. Medical Doctors (M.D.s)
   b. Medical Clinics
   c. Mobile Narcotic Treatment Centers
   d. Physician Assistants

5. You work in a community pharmacy across the street from a large teaching hospital. You receive a prescription for Percocet written for a 12-year-old child who was seen in the emergency room of the hospital. The prescription is written by Dr. Anh, an internal medicine resident at the hospital, on a hospital prescription pad and has the hospital's DEA number followed by "A16." Assuming there is an exemption from electronic prescription requirements, which of the following are true?
   a. A prescription for Percocet for a 12-year-old child cannot be dispensed.
   b. The prescription is valid but may only be dispensed by the hospital's outpatient pharmacy.
   c. The A16 is an indication that only a quantity of 16 may be dispensed.
   d. The prescription may be filled at your pharmacy.

6. CSOS Signing Certificates are issued to
   a. The pharmacy holding the DEA registration
   b. The pharmacist-in-charge
   c. The DEA registrant (owner) or person who has Power of Attorney
   d. The head of IT security at a pharmacy

7. Main Street Hospital Pharmacy has three areas where IVs are mixed: a suite in the main pharmacy consisting of an anteroom and a positive pressure buffer room where nonhazardous sterile preparations are mixed; a suite in the oncology unit with an anteroom and a negative pressure buffer room where hazardous sterile preparations are mixed; and a segregated compounding area (SCA) in the Surgical Services pharmacy satellite. Which areas need to be ISO 7?
   a. Anteroom in the main pharmacy and anteroom in the oncology unit
   b. Negative pressure buffer room and segregated compounding area
   c. Positive pressure buffer room and negative pressure buffer room
   d. Anteroom in the main pharmacy and negative pressure buffer room

8. Which of the following USP chapters have been adopted by the Florida Board of Pharmacy? **Select all that apply.**
   a. Chapter 85, Endotoxins Test
   b. Chapter 731, Loss on Drying
   c. Chapter 797, Pharmaceutical Compounding—Sterile Products
   d. Chapter 800, Hazardous Drugs

9. Pharmacist Pat is compounding eye drops from conventionally manufactured cefazolin injection and artificial tears. Which USP Chapters apply when compounding this preparation?
   a. USP 795
   b. USP 797
   c. USP 800
   d. USP 825

10. Pharmacist Kurt reconstitutes a pharmacy bulk package of vancomycin to make a batch of 10 IV bags for dispensing today. What is the risk level of the batch of preparations he is compounding?
    a. Immediate Use
    b. Low Risk
    c. Medium Risk
    d. High Risk

11. A pharmacist in Tampa receives an electronic prescription from an emergency room physician for 17-year-old Amanda Smith, who was admitted to the emergency room for a kidney stone. The prescription is for 21 tablets of Percocet with instructions to take 1 tablet every 8 hours for pain. Prior to filling the prescription, the pharmacist attempts to check the Prescription Drug Monitoring System, but an afternoon thunderstorm has temporarily knocked out access to the system. Which of the following is true?
    a. The pharmacist may dispense the entire 7-day supply if she documents the reason the PDMP was not checked.
    b. The pharmacist may dispense a 3-day supply if she documents the reason the PDMP was not checked.
    c. The pharmacist may not dispense Percocet to a 17-year-old under these circumstances.
    d. The pharmacist must wait until the PDMP system is operational before dispensing any part of the prescription.

12. Pharmacist Ed receives a prescription for Hycodan Cough Syrup for a patient being treated for an unrelenting cough. The instructions for use are to take 5 ml every 6 hours for the cough. What is the maximum quantity that can be prescribed and dispensed?
    a. 60 ml
    b. 140 ml if the prescriber wrote "Acute Pain Exception" on Rx
    c. 600 ml
    d. There is no legal limit on the quantity

13. A prescriber is treating a patient following an automobile accident, and the patient has an Injury Severity Score of greater than 9. Which of the following must the prescriber do in order to prescribe more than a 7-day supply of a Schedule II opioid? **Select all that apply.**
    a. Write the words "Acute Pain Exception" on the prescription.
    b. Write the words "Nonacute Pain" on the prescription.
    c. Write the words "Traumatic Injury" on the prescription.
    d. Issue an additional prescription for emergency naloxone.

14. Which of the following persons are eligible to serve on the Florida Board of Pharmacy? **Select all that apply.**
    a. Frank Ferlita, a pharmacist licensed in Florida since 2010 who works for a chain pharmacy and lives in Atlanta, Georgia.
    b. Wilma Wallace, a pharmacist in Tampa, Florida, who has been practicing in a hospice pharmacy since 2011.
    c. Bill Politico, a real estate lawyer in West Palm Beach, Florida, who has no affiliation with the practice of pharmacy.
    d. Norma Rios, a pharmacy technician living in Chipley, Florida, who has been a registered pharmacy technician in Florida since 2014 and works in a hospital pharmacy.

15. Pharmacist Bill orders and receives a bottle of generic glipizide from his supplier. Bill notices the label of the bottle is crooked and some of the lettering on the label appears to have different fonts in the same word. Bill calls the supplier to verify the transaction data and learns that the lot number on the bottle is not a valid lot number for that brand of glipizide. What is Bill required to do? **Select all that apply.**
    a. Notify FDA and all trading partners of this illegitimate product.
    b. Take steps to work with the manufacturer to prevent the illegitimate product from reaching patients.
    c. Order a Class I recall of the drug.
    d. Notify DEA.

16. Which of the following is not required on the label of an OTC product?
    a. Adequate directions for safe and effective use
    b. Name and address of the manufacturer, packager, or distributor
    c. Inactive ingredients
    d. NDC number

17. Which of the following is true regarding DEA Form 106?
    a. It should be used to document waste of a controlled substance.
    b. It must be signed by two witnesses.
    c. It must be sent to DEA within one business day of discovery of a significant loss or theft of controlled substances.
    d. It may be filled out online.

18. When utilizing a single-copy DEA Form 222 to order Schedule II controlled substances, who is responsible for making a copy of the form?
    a. The supplier
    b. The purchaser
    c. DEA
    d. The PDMP program manager

19. The monthly sales purchase limit for pseudoephedrine products is
    a. 0.6 g of base product
    b. 2.6 g of base product
    c. 3.6 g of base product
    d. 9 g of base product

20. CMS requires that consultant pharmacists perform a medication regimen review for long-term care patients
    a. When requested by the facility
    b. At least weekly
    c. At least every 30 days
    d. When a medication error occurs

21. Dr. Trang calls your pharmacy and asks if she can call in a prescription for Vicodin for Mr. Garcia, a cancer patient who is well known to you. Dr. Trang states that Mr. Garcia cannot get relief from any other pain medication, and that Mr. Garcia is unable to get to her office to pick up a prescription. She asks if you can fill the prescription and deliver it to Mr. Garcia's house. Assuming an exception to the electronic prescription requirement applies, which of the following is true?
    a. You cannot take a verbal prescription for Vicodin under these circumstances because Mr. Garcia is not a hospice patient.
    b. You can take the verbal prescription, but Dr. Trang must send you a written or electronic prescription for the Vicodin within 7 days.
    c. You can take the verbal prescription and fill the prescription, but it can only be for a 72-hour supply.
    d. Both b and c

22. Which of the following drugs may be prescribed by a DATA-waived practitioner for treatment of narcotic addiction? **Select all that apply.**
    a. Buprenorphine
    b. Naloxone
    c. Buprenorphine/Naloxone combination
    d. Methadone

23. Pharmacist Phil owns and operates Phil's Pills, an independent community pharmacy in Indian Rocks Beach, Florida. Phil has regular seasonal customers, including Mrs. Winston, who just arrived to spend the winter months in Florida. Mrs. Winston brought in written prescriptions from her physician in New Jersey for the following:

    Losartan 50 mg daily, #90, 0 refills
    Glipizide 2.5 mg every morning #90, 0 refills

    When she got to the pharmacy, she remembered she should also have a prescription for Eliquis 2.5 mg daily and asks Phil to call her physician in New Jersey to get a prescription for a 3-month supply of the Eliquis.

    What can Phil do?
    a. Phil cannot fill any of Mrs. Winston's prescriptions because her physician is from out of state.
    b. Phil can fill the two written prescriptions but cannot fill a verbal prescription for Eliquis from a physician in New Jersey.
    c. Phil can fill the two written prescriptions and call to get a verbal prescription for Eliquis and fill all three prescriptions.
    d. Phil can fill the two written prescriptions and call to get the prescription for Eliquis, but it must be limited to a 30-day supply.

24. Who is responsible for determining the contents of an Emergency Drug Kit in a nursing home? **Select all that apply.**
    a. Consultant pharmacist
    b. Facility Medical Director
    c. Facility Director of Nursing
    d. Formulary Committee

25. When dispensing a Customized Medication Package to a patient, the beyond-use date may not exceed
    a. 30 days
    b. 60 days
    c. 90 days
    d. One year

26. St. Mary's Central Hospital is located in Jacksonville, Florida, and provides comprehensive health services to the community through the main hospital and two affiliated hospitals, St. Mary's Riverside and St. Mary's Northside. As the Director of Pharmacy, you have been asked to set up a drug prepackaging operation at St. Mary's Central Hospital that will provide centralized distribution of the prepackaged drugs and IV products to the other two hospitals. Which permit is required for St. Mary's Central Hospital in order to do this?
    a. Class I Institutional
    b. Class II Institutional
    c. Class III Institutional
    d. Special Central Distribution

27. Which of the following products may be ordered and dispensed to a patient by a pharmacist in Florida? **Select all that apply.**
    a. Scopolamine patch
    b. Testosterone topical gel
    c. Erythromycin topical gel
    d. Triamcinolone 0.5% ointment

28. Which of the following is not required on a prescription label?
    a. Name of the drug dispensed
    b. Directions for use
    c. Name of the prescriber
    d. Address of the prescriber

29. For which of the following products is generic substitution prohibited?
    a. Thorazine
    b. Synthroid
    c. Digoxin
    d. Coumadin

30. Put the following in order from shortest time to longest time.
    a. Time limit to receive a written or electronic prescription from a prescriber after accepting an emergency verbal prescription for a Schedule II controlled substance.
    b. Time limit to notify the county sheriff of a person attempting to obtain controlled substances by fraud that occurs on a Monday morning.
    c. Maximum time allowed to print out a hard copy of a pharmacy's dispensing information from the computer upon request from the Department of Health to avoid a finding of failure to maintain records.
    d. Time limit for obtaining all partial refills on a Schedule II prescription when the partial fill was requested by the patient.

31. A Class II institutional pharmacy that also has a Special Sterile Compounding Permit has two pharmacists on duty at all times. One pharmacist supervises pharmacy technicians in the IV room while the other pharmacist manages the other aspects of the pharmacy, including supervising those pharmacy technicians not compounding sterile products. What is the maximum number of pharmacy technicians that can be working at one time at the pharmacy?
    a. 3
    b. 6
    c. 9
    d. 12

32. Bill Ward practiced at and owned City Drug, a pharmacy in Miami, for 15 years with no negative action taken against his license or the pharmacy permit. Unfortunately, after getting mixed up in an illegal compounding scheme involving pain creams, he faced criminal charges. He hired a good lawyer and got the criminal charges dismissed, but his pharmacist license was suspended for six months. The pharmacy permit for City Drug was also revoked. When can Bill apply to the Board of Pharmacy to open a new pharmacy as an owner?
    a. Bill is not eligible to apply for a new pharmacy permit as an owner.
    b. Bill can apply for a pharmacy permit after his six-month suspension is over.
    c. Bill must wait at least 1 year from the date of the pharmacy permit revocation before applying for a pharmacy permit as an owner.
    d. Bill must wait at least 5 years from the date of the pharmacy permit revocation before applying for a pharmacy permit as an owner.

33. For which of the following violations may the Board issue a citation for a first-time offense? **Select all that apply.**
    a. Operating a pharmacy with an inactive permit.
    b. Failure to consult the PDMP prior to dispensing a controlled substance prescription.
    c. Failure to meet the required continuing education requirements.
    d. Dispensing a prescription drug based on a communication that purports to be a prescription when the pharmacist has reason to believe it is not based on a valid practitioner-patient relationship.

34. How many hours of the required continuing education needed to renew a pharmacist's license must be for live seminars, video conferences, or interactive computer-based applications?
    a. 3 hours
    b. 5 hours
    c. 10 hours
    d. 20 hours

35. How many hours of consultant pharmacist continuing education are required for a consultant pharmacist to renew their license?
    a. 15 hours
    b. 24 hours
    c. 30 hours
    d. 45 hours

36. Holiday Regional Hospital is a full-service hospital providing comprehensive medical care to patients in the area. The hospital pharmacy provides the following services from the facility:

    Inpatient pharmacy services including compounding of sterile pharmaceuticals
    Outpatient pharmacy services for employees and medical staff only

    Which pharmacy permits must Holiday Regional Hospital obtain? **Select all that apply.**
    a. Class II Institutional
    b. Special—Limited Community
    c. Special—Parenteral/Enteral Extended Scope
    d. Special—Sterile Compounding

37. Will and Martha Russell and their twins David and Allison (age 16) have been long-time customers of your pharmacy and are planning a trip to Bhutan. They have requested you to provide each of them with a Typhoid vaccine before their trip. Which of the following statements are true?
   a. You cannot provide Typhoid vaccines under a protocol to patients.
   b. You may provide Typhoid vaccines to Will and Martha if it is included in your protocol, but you cannot provide a Typhoid vaccine to David and Allison.
   c. You may provide Typhoid vaccines if it is included in your protocol for all the family members.
   d. You can provide Typhoid vaccines to all family members only if they sign a waiver of liability form.

38. When a central fill pharmacy fills prescriptions for an originating pharmacy, what is required to be on the label?
   a. Only the name of the central fill pharmacy
   b. Only the name of the originating pharmacy
   c. Both pharmacies must be identified on the label, but the originating pharmacy may be identified by a code.
   d. Both pharmacies must be identified on the label, but the central fill pharmacy may be identified by a code.

39. What is the minimum number of hours that a community pharmacy must be open?
   a. 15 hours per week
   b. 20 hours per week
   c. 30 hours per week
   d. 40 hours per week

40. All original prescriptions must be maintained for
   a. 2 years from the date first dispensed
   b. 2 years from the date of the last filling
   c. 4 years from the date first dispensed
   d. 4 years from the date of the last filling

41. Mrs. Williams is one of your regular customers. She has a history of atrial fibrillation and has been taking amiodarone for the past 6 months. She calls you to request a refill of her amiodarone prescription. You note that there are no refills remaining, but tell Mrs. Williams you will call for a refill authorization. You try calling her physician but cannot get anyone to return your call. You try three additional times and still cannot get anyone to return your calls. Mrs. Williams comes to your pharmacy later that day and informs you she is completely out of amiodarone. Which of the following statements are true?
   a. You cannot legally provide Mrs. Williams with a refill, but given the situation you should provide her a 3-day supply.
   b. You cannot legally provide Mrs. Williams with a refill, but given the situation you should provide her a 30-day supply.
   c. You can legally provide Mrs. Williams with an emergency refill of a 3-day supply in this situation.
   d. You can legally provide Mrs. Williams with an emergency refill of a 30-day supply in this situation.

42. What type of drugs may be returned to a closed-door pharmacy and be re-dispensed?
   a. No drugs may be returned to a pharmacy and be re-dispensed.
   b. All unused drugs
   c. All unused drugs in unit-dose or customized medication packages
   d. All unused non-controlled drugs
   e. All unused non-controlled drugs in unit-dose or customized medication packages

43. A medication that has a low risk of drug allergy, drug interaction, dosing error, or adverse patient outcomes, and may be removed and administered from an automated distribution system without a prospective drug use review, is called
   a. An override medication
   b. A low-risk medication
   c. A low-risk override medication
   d. A physician-controlled medication

44. Your pharmacy has been asked to provide an Emergency Medication Kit for a nursing home. Which of the following statements are true?
   a. An inventory of the drugs in the Emergency Medication Kit must be attached to the outside of the kit.
   b. A pharmacy may provide an Emergency Medication Kit to a nursing home, but the kit may not contain any controlled substances.
   c. A pharmacy may only provide an Emergency Medication Kit to a nursing home if the drugs are stored in an automated dispensing machine.
   d. Only a Class I pharmacy may supply an Emergency Medication Kit to a nursing home.

45. When a pharmacist goes on a meal break, which of the following activities may a registered pharmacy technician perform?
   a. Data entry on a new prescription
   b. Conduct a drug regimen review on a refill prescription
   c. Take a new verbal prescription
   d. None of the above

46. A fire broke out in the front part of Debra's pharmacy, but the flames did not reach the prescription department. Can Debra still dispense the drugs?
   a. Yes, as long as the containers are all closed.
   b. Yes, unless the drugs are heat sensitive.
   c. Yes, but only after notifying patients that their prescription may have been exposed to smoke.
   d. No, the smoke from the fire may have adulterated the drugs.

47. What must be provided prior to the first dose and every 30 days thereafter to a patient in an institutional setting who is taking an estrogen prescription?
   a. A safety data sheet
   b. A package insert
   c. A patient package insert
   d. A Medication Guide

48. Anabolic steroids are classified under which schedule?
   a. Schedule II
   b. Schedule III
   c. Schedule IV
   d. Schedule V
   e. None of the above

49. A pharmacist receives a written prescription for fentanyl patches. The pharmacist consults with the prescriber of the medication. After such consultation, which of the following pieces of information may not be changed on the prescription even if the prescriber authorizes the change?
   a. Patient's address
   b. Patient's name
   c. Drug strength
   d. Drug quantity
   e. Directions for use

50. For which class of recall is there a reasonable probability that the product could cause serious adverse effects or death?
   a. Class I
   b. Class II
   c. Class III
   d. Class IV

51. Which of the following is NOT a permissible use or disclosure of protected health information under HIPAA?
   a. Providing a list of all prescription medications to a patient's primary care physician
   b. Sending prescription information to a third-party insurance company for payment purposes
   c. Sending coupons for diapers to all pharmacy customers taking prenatal vitamins
   d. Providing a face-to-face recommendation of an OTC product to a patient based on the patient's symptoms and drug allergy profile

52. If a supplier cannot provide the entire quantity of a Schedule II controlled substance ordered on a DEA Form 222, the remaining quantity must be sent
   a. Within 72 hours
   b. Within 7 days
   c. Within 30 days
   d. Within 60 days

53. How many consumer members serve on the Florida Board of Pharmacy?
    a. 1
    b. 2
    c. 3
    d. 5

54. How can a prescriber legally prohibit generic substitution on a written prescription?
    a. By checking the "dispense as written" box
    b. By writing the words "dispense as written"
    c. By signing the prescription on the "dispense as written" signature line
    d. By writing the words "medically necessary"
    e. All of the above

55. A medium-risk compounded sterile product for which you do not have stability information that is stored in a refrigerator may be assigned a beyond-use date of
    a. 48 hours
    b. 3 days
    c. 9 days
    d. 45 days

56. A nuclear pharmacist must obtain how many additional hours of internship related to radiopharmaceuticals and nuclear pharmacy?
    a. 200 hours
    b. 500 hours
    c. 750 hours
    d. 1,080 hours

57. After an investigation, the Department of Health will make a recommendation to either dismiss a complaint or file an administrative complaint. That recommendation is made to:
    a. The Pharmacy Disciplinary Committee of the Florida Board of Pharmacy
    b. The prosecuting attorney for the Florida Board of Pharmacy
    c. The Probable Cause Committee of the Florida Board of Pharmacy
    d. The Executive Director of the Florida Board of Pharmacy

58. Which type of facility is likely to have a Modified Class II Institutional Pharmacy Permit?
   a. A central fill pharmacy
   b. A remote order entry pharmacy
   c. A teaching hospital
   d. A freestanding emergency room

59. In a community pharmacy, prospective drug use review must be conducted
   a. On all new and refill prescriptions
   b. On new prescriptions, but not refills
   c. When necessary in the professional judgment of the pharmacist
   d. Whenever the computer system flags a potential problem with a prescription

60. What is the maximum amount of a Schedule V product containing codeine that a patient can purchase without a prescription in any 48-hour period?
   a. 60 mg or 60 cc (2 oz.)
   b. 120 mg or 120 cc (4 oz.)
   c. 240 mg or 240 cc (8 oz.)
   d. Patients cannot purchase Schedule V codeine products without a prescription in Florida.

EXPLANATORY ANSWERS

1. C.
This law went into effect July 1, 2020, and requires a pharmacist to complete an initial training course of 20 hours in order to enter into a collaborative practice agreement with a physician. With each renewal, there is a requirement for an 8-hour course. There are several other requirements outlined in the law.

2. B. and C.
The test and treat law allows a certified pharmacist to test and treat for minor, non-chronic health conditions. The law specifically includes streptococcus and lice.

3. B.
Always check to be sure the narcotic substance— in this question, codeine—is being compounded with another therapeutic ingredient first because if it is not, the answer will be Schedule II regardless of the concentration. In this case, the codeine is being compounded with acetaminophen, so you do need to calculate the concentration of codeine. 16mg/5ml (teaspoon) = 320mg/100ml. This is greater than the maximum concentration for Schedule V of 200mg/ml and less than the maximum concentration for Schedule III of 1.8g/100ml, so this is a Schedule III prescription.

4. D.
The M in the first part of a DEA registration stands for "mid-level practitioner," and a physician assistant is a type of mid-level practitioner.

5. D.
An intern or resident in a hospital can issue controlled substance prescriptions using the hospital's DEA registration as long as it is for a patient that was treated at the hospital and the hospital uses a code or suffix on the DEA number to identify who the prescriber is. That is the A16 in this question. These prescriptions are valid and can be dispensed by any pharmacy, not just the hospital outpatient pharmacy.

6. C.
CSOS Signing Certificates are not assigned to the pharmacy, they are assigned to individuals. They can only be issued to the registrant, which in the case of a pharmacy would be the owner if it is a sole proprietor, a partner if it is a partnership, or a corporate officer if it is a corporation. They can also be issued to any individual who has a Power of Attorney to order Schedule II controlled substances.

7. C.
Areas that must be ISO 7 or cleaner are buffer rooms (both positive and negative pressure) and anterooms that open into a negative pressure room. Anterooms that open only into positive pressure buffer rooms must be at least ISO 8. Segregated compounding areas do not need to be ISO classified.

8. A., B., and C.
Florida has adopted the following USP Chapters: Chapter 797—Pharmaceutical Compounding—Sterile Preparations, Chapter 71—Sterility Tests, Chapter 85—Bacterial Endotoxins Test, and Chapter 731—Loss on Drying. USP Chapter 800 has not been adopted by the Florida Board of Pharmacy, but is included in this review because it is mentioned in the MPJE Competency Statements.

9. B.
Ophthalmics—including drops—need to be sterile, so USP 797 applies. Cefazolin is not a hazardous drug, so 800 does not apply in this case.

10. C.
A pharmacy bulk package is a conventionally manufactured dosage form. Any batch product compounded from all sterile components is a medium-risk preparation.

11. B.
Although checking of the PDMP is mandatory, there are specific situations where it is not required, including when the system is not operating. For any of those situations, the law limits the amount that can be prescribed or dispensed to a 3-day supply and requires documentation of the reason why the PDMP was not checked.

12. D.

   Hycodan Cough Syrup contains hydrocodone bitartrate and is a Schedule II controlled substance. However, it is not being prescribed for acute pain; it is being prescribed for cough. The Florida days' supply limit would not apply in this case, and there is not a days' supply limit on a single prescription for a controlled substance. Of course, a pharmacist would need to use professional judgment, but legally there is no days' supply limit.

13. B. and D.

   A traumatic injury with an Injury Severity Score of 9 or greater is, by definition, not acute pain. In order to prescribe more than a 7-day supply of an opioid, a prescriber must write "Non-acute pain" on the prescription. For traumatic injuries with an Injury Severity Score of 9 or greater, there is an additional requirement to prescribe an emergency opioid antagonist. The phrase "Acute Pain Exception" is used to prescribe a 7-day supply instead of a 3-day supply, but that does not apply to this situation.

14. B. and C.

   Both pharmacist members and consumer members of the Board of Pharmacy must be residents of Florida. Pharmacist members must also have been engaged in the practice of pharmacy for at least 4 years. Consumer members may not be connected with the pharmacy profession, a drug manufacturer, or drug wholesaler.

15. A. and B.

   Under the Drug Supply Chain Security Act, a pharmacy that identifies an illegitimate product must notify FDA using Form FDA 3911, notify trading partners within 24 hours, and work with the manufacturer to prevent the illegitimate product from reaching patients. While a recall may be necessary, that responsibility would normally fall on the manufacturer.

16. D.

   Although NDC numbers are required in order for manufacturers to list their drug products with the FDA, they are technically not required on the label. All of the other items are required elements on an OTC drug label.

17. D.

The DEA 106 form is used to document a theft or significant loss of controlled substances. While an initial notice to the DEA must be made within one business day of discovery, this does not mean the DEA 106 form has to be completed by then. A pharmacist may need time to investigate the extent and scope of the theft or loss because the DEA 106 form requires listing each controlled substance that was lost or stolen, and that may take some time. No witnesses are required to sign the DEA 106 form.

18. B.

When utilizing a single-copy DEA 222 form, the purchaser must make a copy of the form. This is necessary because the form is used to document the Schedule II drugs that are later received in the pharmacy. With the triplicate DEA 222 form, the purchaser keeps copy 3, where the receipt of the drugs is indicated, so it makes sense that with a single-copy form, the purchaser would need to make a copy before sending it to the supplier.

19. C.

The Combat Methamphetamine Epidemic Act limits the retail purchase of pseudoephedrine products to 3.6 g of the base product per day and 9 g of the base product per 30 days. The electronic system used in pharmacies monitors for total purchases by each purchaser's driver's license to prevent purchases that exceed these amounts, so this is not something most pharmacists have to know or calculate, but you need to know these limits for the MPJE.

20. C.

CMS regulations require a consultant pharmacist to perform a medication regimen review for LTCS patients every 30 days. This is one of the few CMS rules that impact pharmacy practice directly, and it is included in the MPJE competencies.

21. D.

Both Florida and federal law permit verbal prescriptions for Schedule II controlled substance in an emergency, and this fact situation qualifies as an emergency. There is no requirement that the patient be in hospice. Both Florida law and federal law require the prescriber to send an electronic or written controlled substance to the pharmacy within 7 days after authorizing an emergency dispensing of a Schedule II controlled substance. Florida restricts the amount that can be dispensed in this situation to a 72-hour supply.

22. A. and C.
DATA-waived practitioners can only prescribe two drugs to treat opioid addiction: buprenorphine and buprenorphine/naloxone combination. Methadone is used to treat opioid addiction, but it cannot be prescribed or dispensed for this purpose.

23. C.
Prescriptions from out-of-state practitioners are valid in Florida if for the treatment of a chronic or recurrent illness. These prescriptions may be electronic, written, or verbal. The mandatory electronic requirements do not apply to out-of-state practitioners, as they are not licensed in Florida. There is no 30-day supply limit for the verbal prescription because Eliquis is not a Schedule III drug.

24. A., B., and C.
Florida law does not specify which drugs may be placed in an Emergency Medication Kit, but it allows each facility to make that determination. Specifically, the rule requires the contents of the Emergency Drug Kit to be determined by the facility's medical director, the director of nursing, and the consultant pharmacist.

25. B.
Customized Medication Packages contain two or more solid oral dosage forms packaged in a manner to improve patient compliance with drug therapy. These packages may not have a beyond-use date that exceeds 60 days.

26. C.
Institutional Class I pharmacy permits are generally for nursing homes. A hospital pharmacy normally has an Institutional Class II pharmacy permit. However, if a hospital is prepackaging drugs for use at affiliated facilities, they would need an Institutional Class III permit.

27. A. and C.
Even though the law allowing pharmacists to order and dispense certain medicinal drugs is not used in practice very often, it is unique to Florida and is still in place, so you should be familiar with the formulary of drugs authorized and the requirements for this practice.

28. D.

The address of the prescriber is not required to be placed on the label of a prescription drug. You should know all of the labeling requirements for prescription drugs.

29. A.

Thorazine is the brand name for chlorpromazine and is included on the negative formulary in Florida and cannot be substituted. Digoxin is not on the negative formulary; digitoxin is included, but this product is no longer available in the U.S. Levothyroxine products such as Synthroid were on the negative formulary at one time but were later removed. You should memorize all of the drugs on the negative formulary.

30. B., C., A., and D.

B = Within 24 hours or next business day.
C = Within 72 hours of request.
A = Within 7 days.
D = 30 days.

31. C.

Because pharmacy technicians are involved in sterile compounding, the ratio of pharmacists to technicians for that part of the facility is 3:1. Since there is another pharmacist supervising pharmacy technicians in a separate part of the facility (i.e., outside of the IV room), a 6:1 ratio applies there, so the total number of pharmacy technicians allowed is 9.

32. C.

After a pharmacy permit is revoked, the person who owned the pharmacy may not apply for a permit to operate a pharmacy for one year from the date of the revocation.

33. A., B., and C.

Citations are not considered disciplinary action and can be issued for first-time offenses of fairly minor violations, including operating a pharmacy with an inactive permit, failing to consult the PDMP prior to dispensing a controlled substance prescription, and failing to meet the required continuing education requirements.

34. C.
Of the required 30 hours of continuing education, at least 10 hours must be from live seminars, video teleconferences, or interactive computer-based applications.

35. B.
To renew a consultant pharmacist, 24 hours of consultant pharmacist continuing education must be completed. These hours are in addition to the 30 hours to renew a pharmacist license.

36. A., B., and D.
As a hospital providing inpatient services, an Institutional Class II permit is required. Because this hospital is also dispensing outpatient prescriptions for employees and medical staff, a Special—Limited Community Pharmacy permit is also required. A Special—Sterile Products permit is also required because the hospital is compounding sterile products.

37. B.
Florida permits pharmacists and interns who are certified to provide immunizations in the Adult Immunization Schedule of the CDC and those recommended for international travel, but does not permit vaccinations or immunizations by pharmacists or interns to patients under age 18.

38. D.
Both the originating pharmacy and the central fill pharmacy must be identified on a prescription filled via central fill, but the central fill pharmacy may be identified by a code rather than a name and address.

39. B.
A community pharmacy must be opened a minimum of 20 hours per week.

40. D.
All original prescription records must be kept for no less than 4 years from the date of last filling.

41. C.
A onetime emergency refill of up to a 72-hour supply may be provided if a pharmacist is unable to contact the prescriber to obtain authorization for a refill.

42. E.
The exception that allows the return and reuse of drugs in a closed-drug delivery system is limited to drugs that are in unit-dose or customized medication packages and is only permitted for non-controlled substances.

43. C.
Medication with a low risk of drug allergy, drug interaction, dosing error, or adverse patient outcome is known as a low-risk override medication and may be removed from an automated distribution system without a prospective drug use review by a pharmacist.

44. A.
An Emergency Medication Kit must have an inventory of its contents attached to the outside of the kit. Florida does not restrict the types or quantities of the drugs that may be stored in an emergency kit. While an automated dispensing machine may be used as an Emergency Medication Kit, there is not a requirement that one be used.

45. A.
When a pharmacist is on a meal break, pharmacy technicians may stay in the pharmacy and perform technician duties such as prescription data entry. A pharmacy technician can never perform prospective drug use review or take new verbal prescriptions.

46. D.
A drug does not have to be contaminated to be adulterated. If it was held under conditions where it may have been contaminated, it is considered adulterated. Because there was a fire and smoke in the pharmacy, the drugs in the pharmacy may have been contaminated and are therefore adulterated.

47. C.
A patient package insert must be provided to institutionalized patients prior to the first dose and every 30 days thereafter for estrogen-containing drugs and oral contraceptives.

48. B.
Anabolic steroids are classified as Schedule III controlled substances.

49. B.
On a written Schedule II controlled substance prescription, a pharmacist may call to change most items and document those changes on the prescription, but cannot do that for the name of the patient, name of the drug, name of the prescriber, and date.

50. A.
A Class A recall is one where there is a reasonable probability that the product could cause serious adverse effects or death.

51. C.
Sending coupons for diapers to all pharmacy customers taking prenatal vitamins is using patients' protected health information (PHI) to market another product and is not permissible under HIPAA without the consent of the patients. All of the other choices fit into the exceptions for payment, treatment, or healthcare operations.

52. D.
A supplier may provide a partial quantity of an order for Schedule II controlled substances on a DEA Form 222 and has 60 days to send the remaining quantity.

53. B.
The Florida Board of Pharmacy has 2 consumer members.

54. D.
A prescriber can legally prohibit generic substitution on a written prescription by writing the words "brand medically necessary."

55. C.
Medium-risk sterile products that are stored under refrigeration may be assigned a beyond-use date of 9 days. It is recommended that you memorize the maximum beyond-use dates for different risk levels and storage conditions.

56. B.
Nuclear pharmacists must complete a radiopharmacy internship of at least 500 hours.

57. C.
Recommendations to either dismiss a complaint or file an administrative complaint are made by the Probable Cause Committee of the Board of Pharmacy.

58. D.
Short-term primary care treatment centers that meet all of the requirements for an Institutional Class II permit, except space and equipment requirements such as free-standing emergency rooms, are permitted as Modified Class II Institutional Pharmacies.

59. A.
Prospective drug use review in a community pharmacy is required for all new and refill prescriptions.

60. B.
Even though this is not done in practice very often, you need to know the requirements and limitations for dispensing Schedule V controlled substances without a prescription. For codeine, the maximum quantity in a 48-hour time period is 120 mg.